D1765890

Live
Stronger
Live
Longer

Dedication

*This book is dedicated
to all those people
whose brains wrote cheques
their body couldn't cash.*

DR MARK AWERBUCH

FRCP, FFPMANZCA

Live Stronger Live Longer

*An exercise and lifestyle program
for over 40s*

Sydney New York St.Louis San Francisco Auckland Bogotá
Caracas Lisbon London Madrid MexicoCity Milan Montreal
New Delhi SanJuan Singapore Tokyo Toronto

Reprinted 2002
Text © 2001 Mark Awerbuch
Illustrations and design © 2001 McGraw-Hill Australia Pty Ltd
Additional owners of copyright are named in on-page credits.

Apart from any fair dealing for the purposes of study, research, criticism or review, as
permitted under the *Copyright Act*, no part may be reproduced by any process without
written permission. Enquiries should be made to the publisher, marked for the attention
of the Permissions Editor, at the address below.

Every effort has been made to trace and acknowledge copyright material. Should any
infringement have occurred accidentally the authors and publishers tender their
apologies.

Copying for educational purposes
Under the copying provisions of the Copyright Act, copies of parts of this book may be
made by an educational institution. An agreement exists between the Copyright Agency
Limited (CAL) and the relevant educational authority (Department of Education,
university, TAFE, etc.) to pay a licence fee for such copying. It is not necessary to keep
records of copying except where the relevant educational authority has undertaken to do
so by arrangement with the Copyright Agency Limited.

For further information on the CAL licence agreements with educational institutions, ·
contact the Copyright Agency Limited, Level 19, 157 Liverpool Street, Sydney NSW 2000.
Where no such agreement exists, the copyright owner is entitled to claim payment
in respect of any copies made.

Enquiries concerning copyright in McGraw-Hill publications should be directed to the
Permissions Editor at the address below.

National Library of Australia Cataloguing-in-Publication data:

Awerbuch, Mark
Live stronger, live longer : a lifestyle program for over 40s and people with arthritis.

Includes index.
ISBN 0 074 71087 7.

1.Weight training. 2. Physical fitness. 3. Arthritis – Prevention.
4. Aging – Prevention. I. Title.

613.713

Published in Australia by
McGraw-Hill Australia Pty Ltd
4 Barcoo Street, Roseville NSW 2069, Australia
Acquisitions Editor: Meiling Voon
Production Editor: Megan Lowe
Editor: Michael Wall
Designer (cover and interior): Norman Baptista
Typeset in Palatino by Norman Baptista
Printed on 80 gsm woodfree by Ligare Pty. Ltd., Australia.

Comments about the book

'...this is not just an exercise book, it's a whole of life book—it provides sensible advice on nutrition and on simple exercises that you can do at home or in a gymnasium. The advice is sensible and more than that, it's achievable.'

Professor Peter Brooks
National Co-ordinator, Australian Federal Government
Bone and Joint Decade Initiative

'*Live Stronger Live Longer* is a genuinely inspirational book offering for the first time a winning lifestyle formula for everyone willing to give it a go.'

Gary Player
US and British Open Golfing Champion

'We would like to applaud your book *Live Stronger Live Longer* and your personal commitment to supporting older people to improve their strength, fitness, well-being and their quality of life.'

Patricia Reeve
Executive Director, Council on the Ageing Victoria

'...an outstanding lifestyle program for anyone over 40.'

Shaun Tomson
World Surfing Champion

'...this book will be one of the shining pointers for those who wish to help themselves. I think that more importantly than prolonging life, the feeling of fitness will make life so much more enjoyable. I will unhesitatingly recommend this book to patients and friends.'

Dr Julian de Jager
President, Australian Rheumatology Association

'As a person with Arthritis and also a great believer in exercise, I wholeheartedly endorse your program which simplifies the issues and provides an easy to follow system for the over 40s.'

Barry Richards
World Series Cricketer

'This book should inspire older people to take care of themselves by regular exercise and sensible eating.'

Phil Rabinowitz
World's Oldest Competitive Walker of Over 20 km events,
Guinness Book of World Records
(completed Sydney's 14 km City to Surf Run at 97 years old)

Foreword

Having recognised the alternative, most people accept old age as one of life's inevitabilities, albeit without much enthusiasm.

As the life expectancy of the population increases, it is up to each of us to ensure that our later years remain active and interesting. The fear of ageing arises from picturing the worst outcomes of infirmity and immobility.

There is no doubt that patterns of activity that provide a mix of aerobic or cardiovascular fitness, muscle toning and joint flexibility will sustain good health, enhance the immune system and reduce the risk of illness. Not all forms of exercise suit everyone, but in *Live Stronger—Live Longer* Mark Awerbuch outlines training programs with an emphasis on safety that have been specifically designed for those of us over the age of 40 and for people with arthritis, irrespective of starting levels of fitness and strength.

After gently convincing the reader of the benefits of adopting an appropriate lifestyle, Mark presents in a clear, detailed but simple way the steps to achieving such outcomes.

Changing a pattern of eating and following an exercise program can be threatening to one's comfort zone. For those who would like to make changes but are uncertain how to get started or how to find an exercise program that is appropriate and safe for their age or particular joint condition, this is the book for you.

Thousands of athletes compete at Olympic Games and we marvel at outstanding gold medal performances or when excellent results are achieved against great odds. The founder of the modern Olympics, Baron de Coubertin, stated that 'The Olympic idea is the conception of a strong physical culture'. He advised that 'the important thing in life is not victory but struggle, the essential is not to have won but to have fought well'.

While only a small percentage of athletes win medals, it is the joy of participation and the achievement of PBs ('personal bests' in athletic parlance) that is most cherished, providing lifelong memories and a sense of satisfaction. Translating this to everyday life, it is not necessary to be the fastest or the strongest in our particular social or age group but to take part, to get involved and to explore our potential. By following the clear directions outlined in this book you can achieve a high level of cardiovascular fitness, muscle strength, joint protection and, importantly, a sense of well being.

The author brings to this book not only the professional skills of a specialist rheumatologist and pain physician but the credibility of personal experience in overcoming the challenges of middle age and joint degeneration through following the very programs outlined in this book.

This very readable book provides the stimulation and inspiration to engage in regular activity. Here is an enjoyable fitness plan that anyone can follow. For those who may not have contemplated weight training before, this book provides a clear, safe and practical guide on how to get started. For those already exercising regularly the book offers opportunities to build on past gains and to achieve fitness and strength levels not previously considered. For everyone, here is a text to provide a balanced exercise program that will provide all-round benefits and limit the ageing process.

The author is to be congratulated in presenting a book that will allow the reader to achieve his or her maximum potential and enjoy a great quality of life.

Dr Brian Sando OAM
Medical Director of the Australian 2000 Olympic Team
Past National President of Sports Medicine Australia

Contents

Part 2
Getting down to it

Preface

The motivation for this book has its roots in my personal interest and involvement in sports and the relatively recent scientific awakening to the health benefits of regular exercise in people with a wide range of medical conditions—obesity, heart disease, high blood pressure, diabetes, osteoporosis, arthritis, fibromyalgia, depression, insomnia and so on. For people who have none of these conditions regular exercise has been shown to significantly reduce the risk of getting them and, importantly, has been shown to reduce the risk of breast, ovarian and bowel cancer.

Up until the age of 40 I enjoyed nothing more than distance running. As a university student I competed in a number of long-distance road races, including two Comrades Marathons (a 90-kilometre race between two towns in South Africa). I never ever won a race but I always finished. By the time I'd reached my mid-forties my knees were creaking and giving way and I was getting more frequent bouts of back pain related to a disease I'd had since a teenager. I couldn't walk in comfort, let alone run. Cartilage surgery was needed in both knees. Unfortunately a common if not invariable outcome of knee cartilage surgery is an earlier onset of osteoarthritis (degenerative joint disease). Running was out and if I wanted to continue to exercise an alternative had to be found. The alternative was resistance training (weight training), through which I was able to control my knee and back pain and embark on an entirely different course that included low-impact cardiovascular training, martial arts and an expanded resistance training program.

My own experience reinforced by a number of compelling scientific studies in highly credentialled international medical journals encouraged me to incorporate exercise advice into treatment programs for my patients with a range of medical disorders. This book is the result.

Acknowledgments

Almost every acknowledgment in every book begins with something like 'no book represents the work of one individual', and so it is here.

I would like to thank my darling wife Jill and my two amazing daughters Nicky and Kerry for their unstinting support, optimism and constructive criticism. A special thanks to Jill for excusing me from weekend garden duties; to my tireless typist Alana Barker who sweated through cutting, pasting, rewrites and tuna sandwiches; and to Liz Runciman, my research assistant, for whom nothing was too much trouble (or if it was she never told me about it).

Particular thanks to those who read some or all of my manuscript and whose advice and counsel have been invaluable: Professor Les Cleland, Director of Rheumatology at the Royal Adelaide Hospital, for his invaluable advice on Omega 3 fats; Dr Manny Noakes, nutritionist at CSIRO, for her comments and advice on the 'Food and diet' and 'The fat story' chapters; Dr Phil Hamdorf, Head and Chief Exercise Physiologist, Centre for Physical Activity in Ageing, Royal Adelaide Hospital, South Australia and President of the Association for Exercise and Sports Science, for his positive comments, help with references and encouragement; Ann Angove, Catherine Davies and Sandra Schirmer of the Muscular Development Fitness Unit, Memorial Hospital, for their tutorial on transversus abdominis, back bracing and resistance band exercises and for their helpful comments on my manuscript.

Others who contributed helpful advice include Dr Ian Hamilton Craig, author of *Cholesterol Control*, Dr John Graham, endocrinologist, Julieanne McKeough, dietitian, Robyn Wall, physiotherapist, and Sandy Frazer, author of *Living Lite*.

Thanks to Paul Frazer of Cut and Paste Studio for photographic work. Special thanks to David Leask of Howden Medical Books, whose kindness and foresight resulted in my association with my publisher, McGraw-Hill.

Over the last 12 years I have had the good fortune and privilege to have learnt from a number of martial artists: Kioshi Gary McRae saw me through to my 1st Dan Black Belt in Zen Do Kai; Matt Michaelis of Xclusive Personal Training taught me kick boxing and fighting technique by, among other things, throwing me into the ring with his security guards, and taught me the benefits of high-intensity 'burnouts', while Naris Lapsis patiently helped me through my katas.

I have also been very fortunate to have found a number of excellent fitness trainers through the years, including Matt Michaelis, Brad Murch, David Wark, Mark Berry and most recently Richard Campbell of the EFM Stirling gym in South Australia, who always gave willingly of his time, knowledge and patience.

A final word of thanks to my brother Brad and to my friends (both in and out of the gym) who, whatever they might have been thinking, provided me with positive input and support.

part 1 Things to be aware of before starting the program

Chapter 1 Making the choice

'It is not good to settle into a set of opinions. It is a mistake to put forth effort and obtain some understanding and then stop at that.'

YAMAMOTO TSUNETOMO
THE BOOK OF THE SAMURAI (HAGAKURE)

This book provides a formula with the potential to improve the quality and the duration of life for people over 40 (including 'baby boomers' like myself) and for people with arthritis, irrespective of age.

It consists of two parts. Part 1 (Chapters 1–10) deals with important safety, dietary and preparatory issues, while Part 2 (Chapters 11–18) sets out a series of exercise programs. You may be tempted to skip Part 1 and cut to the chase, believing that Part 2 is where all the action lies. I encourage you not to do so. Think of yourself as embarking on a new and exciting journey. The success and enjoyment of the journey will to a great extent depend on how well prepared you are for it. This is what Part 1 is about.

The dietary principles in Part 1 and the exercise programs in Part 2 are based on an important piece of scientific knowledge, namely that two-thirds of the ageing process results from lifestyle choices. This is really terrific news and gives cause for tremendous optimism. It puts us in the powerful position of being able to control much of how we will age. There are now compelling scientific data indicating that by modifying lifestyle we can reduce our biological age (the 'actual' age of the cells, tissues, etc.) and live a longer and healthier life. The exercise programs by which we hope to achieve these aims are of two types: resistance (or strength) training, and cardiovascular (endurance/fitness) training.

Anti-ageing medicine is something you might have read or heard about, and speculation is rife about how gene therapy might prolong life. But since only one-third of the ageing process is due to hereditary and biological factors, at best medical science will only ever be able to modify this one-third. We, on the other hand, are in the enviable position of being able to modify *two-thirds* of the ageing process, and we don't have to wait or hope for a new scientific breakthrough. These breakthroughs have already been made and it is on this new science that the programs in this book are based—and you can start as soon as you like.

Some of you over the age of 40 may be wondering why this book is also directed at people with arthritis—what's arthritis got to do with you? Since there is no way of breaking this to you gently, I won't try. The unfortunate reality is that by the time you reach 40 there will be degenerative changes in your joints—even if you've never experienced joint pain. And if you haven't been doing the right exercise you'll have lost muscle, bone and strength as well as flexibility and movement speed. The same thing occurs in younger people who have arthritis.

This knowledge is important. It is our starting point. It underpins the realistic, achievable training programs in this book, which are designed to build muscle and strength, prevent bone loss, restore flexibility and minimise the loss of movement speed. This is something we can do together, and it's fun. At the same time the programs have a 'safety first' policy to minimise the risk of injury and the likelihood of aggravating pre-existing degenerative changes.

Remember we are part of the 'ageing population' we're always reading about, the fastest growing group in today's society. Most of us will live longer than our parents and longer than people in any generation in history. In short we're going to be around a while. The programs outlined in this book are designed to prepare us for a long life, to improve its quality and, with a little bit of luck (and effort), to prolong it.

For me, the inspiration for this book comes from more than 25 years of treating people with arthritis and chronic pain, for many of whom just accomplishing activities of daily living independently is a mini-workout. It's worth noting that almost all of my patients who succeeded in overcoming their individual handicaps have asked the same question: 'What about exercise, doctor?' The resistance training and cardiovascular training programs described in this book are designed to take people with arthritis beyond the point of simply coping independently with daily activities. For those without arthritis the programs are designed to generate a level of strength and fitness in the second half of life to enhance the enjoyment of living and to give substance to the idea that 'life begins at 40'. For those of you who've already achieved a moderate or high level of fitness and strength, the programs offer the opportunity to build on these gains, to explore your potential and, if you wish, to progress to an elite level.

Almost every day of every week people buy lottery tickets in the hope of getting rich. Over a year the average lottery player spends over $500 (and often considerably more) with little to show for it. The mathematical odds of striking a prize that will 'change your life' are, at best, several million to one. Playing the lotteries is like admitting 'I have no control over my life—I want my life enriched by a stroke of luck'. For the same sort of investment you can start a gym program, take control of your life, and enrich it by making your own luck.

It's not just about being active, it's about being *proactive* on the most important issue in your life—your health. It's about doing something decisive before you get the dreaded tap on the shoulder. Setting goals, making commitments and taking responsibility for yourself is a challenge that may at first seem daunting, but being proactive is a lot less daunting than having to be *reactive* after a 'health scare'.

These training programs have been specifically designed to enable over-40-year-olds (whether or not you've had a health scare) and people of all ages with arthritis to achieve personal goals irrespective of baseline strength and fitness levels. The programs neither place unreasonable expectations on you nor seek to impose goals that aren't right for you. They do offer the opportunity to achieve program goals in both strength and cardiovascular fitness, starting at a low intensity (Pre-Level 1 and Level 1), through moderate intensity (Level 2) to high intensity (Level 3), if and when you are ready. The good news is that this is not a lottery. You can succeed whether or not you have arthritis or are just a 40, 50, 60, 70, 80 or 90-year-old who has made up their mind to take control, to fight back.

I ask that you make only one promise—to yourself. Promise yourself to stick with the program for eight weeks. Let this be your first goal. Dropout disease is high within eight weeks of starting any program, but you need at least eight weeks before you start to experience the rewards of your efforts. Once you get to eight weeks you're on your way.

My aim in writing this book is to promote a 'pro-ageing' message in which ageing is seen not as a 'problem' that requires fixing by 'anti-ageing' medicine but as a challenge we can each face up to by adopting a proactive approach to exercise and diet issues. In this way, older adults will not only age successfully but set the pace and act as positive role models for younger people so that we can all be optimistic about the future.

THE BOTTOM LINE

By making a proactive lifestyle choice you can gain control of your life.

Chapter 2

Tackling age
and arthritis

> *'Ageing seems to be the
> only available way to live
> a long time.'*
>
> DANIEL FRANÇOIS ESPRIT AUBER

WHAT'S 'SPECIAL' ABOUT BEING OVER 40?

Well, for one thing you've probably had a big celebration and afterwards wondered, 'What now?', 'Where's it all gone?', or 'What if the next 40 years zoom by just as quickly?' You are not alone!

We all want to live a long life but at the same time we fear old age. There's no need. You can turn this time into something special. After all, we know a whole lot more than we did before. We also know ourselves better—or at least we think we do. I suspect, though, that there are few who *really* know their own physical limits (you'll notice that I didn't say limitations). This is because very few people, apart from elite athletes, have tested or pushed these limits. I'm not going to ask or suggest that you do, because mostly it's not necessary. If you're a baby boomer like me you were probably brought up in an era where the 'no pain no gain' theory ruled. Science has now proved this is not true. Nevertheless it is a misconception that has probably turned off a generation of people who might otherwise have benefited from healthy and enjoyable physical activity.

You may believe that 'resistance training' (weight training) is something done by body builders or at least only by young people. Medical science advises us otherwise. The last 10 years have seen a complete re-evaluation by exercise scientists of the role of resistance training in older adults. A 1990 study demonstrated that resistance training in men and women as old as 90 years resulted in remarkable strength increases—in some cases by more than 100%. Other studies have shown that resistance training in older adults resulted in an increase in strength and endurance, and that the training was *unassociated with any ill effects.*

Some of you reading this may be asking yourselves 'Can I really do this? Am I strong enough to lift weights?' The answer is 'Yes, you are'. Chances are you'll surprise yourself at what you can do. I am not going to ask you to wade into the deep end without first teaching you how to get there and how to stay there safely. *You don't have to be strong to do resistance training. Resistance training will make you strong.*

If you are an older adult or have severe arthritis then initially you may need to begin with low-intensity exercise. This is catered for by the preparatory (Pre-Level 1 and Level 1) training level. Training at these levels for eight to 12 weeks will provide substantial health benefits. Many who start at Pre-Level 1 will, within a short period (often less than six weeks), be able to progress to Level 1 and then further. The moderate-intensity exercise required at Level 2 will take you beyond substantial health benefits to a higher level of strength and fitness. The exercise demands at Level 3 are necessarily of a higher intensity because at this level you are looking to achieve a level of strength and fitness well above the average for your age.

Many people who may not have previously contemplated either resistance training or cardiovascular training may mistakenly believe that those who exercise regularly and who seem to be able to stick to a program week after week are in some way different from themselves. I can tell you that anyone who has exercised regularly has at some time encountered difficulties they've had to overcome, and you too can learn to do this so that you can remain active. In fact the physical differences between individuals are really quite subtle. It may be that at the elite level differences in genetic endowment do make the difference between who gets a gold, silver or bronze medal and who does not, but that's just about it. Mostly it's what people do with *what they have.* The problem is most people don't know what they have.

I went to boarding school at Kearsney College in Botha's Hill, South Africa. The headmaster was Stanley Osler, who in the 1930s had been a rugby Springbok at fly half (five-eighth). Stan was a short, wiry little guy who seemed to bounce off his toes when he walked. As headmaster he wasn't involved in rugby coaching but he'd always come around at training with words of encouragement. Typically he'd look out for the boys who were struggling to keep up or seemed to be doing it tough. Stan's famous saying, which every boy had heard many times over and which he'd say quietly but with conviction, was 'there's more in you yet, laddie, there's more in you yet'. This was an all-boys school but I've no doubt that if it had been co-ed he could just as easily have said 'there's more in you yet, lassie, there's more in you yet'. Of course back then I never believed him and never gave much thought to his words, but they stuck with me and there have since been many times while training or competing when I've 'hit the wall' and had cause to repeat his words and dig that little bit deeper.

DEGENERATIVE JOINT CHANGES

Now, what about those degenerative changes I mentioned earlier? Well, these first appear in our twenties in one of the shoulder joints (the acromioclavicular joint), and by the age of 50 almost all of us will have such changes. By age 40 we'll also have degenerative changes in our elbow tendons and in the rotator cuffs, which hold the shoulder joints in place. Degenerative changes at the base of the neck start to develop in our thirties and, by age 60, 90% of people are affected by this. By age 50, more than 85% of us have X-ray evidence of degenerative changes in the lower back (the lumbar region). And let's not forget the big toe joint. Because this joint carries more weight for its size than any other joint in the body, by age 40, and often much younger, most people have degenerative changes here.

The medical name for these degenerative joint changes is osteoarthritis. Of course many, if not most, of us have no idea these changes have occurred because they're often painless. What *is* important for those of us over 40 is an awareness that these changes are present even when we're pain-free. This knowledge has been carefully considered in creating the training programs in this book. Exercises that pose a risk of injury to vulnerable joints in those over 40 have been modified, but only where this can be done without compromising the benefits of the exercise. Where an exercise cannot be 'made safe' for people in the over-40 age group and for people with arthritis it has been excluded altogether. Fortunately there is a sufficiently wide range of different exercises for the same muscle groups so that it has been possible to find exercises to work all muscle groups without significantly risking joint or tendon injury.

MUSCLE LOSS

There's something else about being 40 or over that's pretty important. This is the age when both men and women start to lose muscle mass. This makes us weaker and less flexible. Consequently we feel like doing less, and we do less. The result is an even greater acceleration of muscle loss and even more weakness. Unfortunately this is also accompanied by an increase in body fat. A vicious cycle has been set up. We have to break out of this downward spiral. This book will show you how.

BONE LOSS

Bone loss, or osteoporosis, is a problem in older men and women, but women are more vulnerable because they start off with thinner bones than men. This becomes an even bigger problem after the menopause because of hormonal changes. Resistance training will significantly reduce the risk of osteoporosis.

LOSS OF FLEXIBILITY

As we get older an alteration takes place in the elasticity of our connective tissue, ligaments and tendons. This adds to the reduction in overall flexibility caused by muscle loss and joint changes. Scientific studies suggest that loss of flexibility is partly due to a reduction in strength and physical activity. Resistance training, which strengthens muscles, together with stretching exercises will improve our flexibility and range of joint movement.

LOSS OF MOVEMENT SPEED
Everyone over 40 years is likely at one time or another to have said either aloud or as a silent curse, 'I'm slowing down'. This is so characteristic of people in their sixties, seventies, eighties and nineties that we think of slowness of movement as an integral and inevitable part of ageing. It happens because of a loss of muscle, bone and flexibility. The resistance training and cardiovascular training programs described in this book will minimise these age effects.

WHAT ABOUT ARTHRITIS?
Arthritis means you have disease of the joints. In some people only a few joints are involved but in others there may be a number of joints affected. These joints hurt when we move them (and sometimes even when we don't) and usually they don't have the same range of movement as normal joints. The result is that they are underused. The result of joint underuse is more than just the obvious loss of range of joint movement. Equally debilitating is the loss of the muscles that normally move the joint accompanied by an overall loss of strength, which leads to an increased risk of falls, bone breaks and a loss of independence. Less well known but equally important is that where joints are moved less the bones themselves become thinner and more liable to break, even after relatively minor trauma. Also, because of underuse you will burn fewer kilojoules (or calories), will gain weight and will place even more stress on your arthritic joints—another debilitating vicious cycle has been established. The programs described in this book will help to break this cycle.

People with arthritis must be growing weary of hearing 'move it or lose it'. Many have already lost a great deal and must wonder what there is left to lose. In fact, as you read this you may be wondering whether resistance training is safe for people with arthritis. You may even be wondering whether you're about to become 'guinea pigs' in a new diabolical experiment. Well, you're not. There are now a number of excellent studies that have documented that resistance training in people with arthritis improves muscle function, stabilises joints, reduces joint load and helps people to better cope with their arthritis. Even more importantly, studies indicate that resistance training can actually improve joint mobility in arthritic joints. However, to avoid potential problems there are a few simple rules and some exercise modifications that people with arthritis will need to follow—these are discussed later in the chapters on modified exercise programs for people with arthritis.

There may be many of you with particular joint impairments requiring specific exercise or equipment modifications to enable you to participate in the resistance training and cardiovascular training programs described in this book. Some of you may have such poor grip strength that you'll have difficulty in holding onto weights, while others may have severe restriction of joint movement, limiting the range through which you can exercise. I'm aware of this. These limitations *can* be accommodated. We *can* work around and through these problems. For example, there are various strap-on ankle and wrist weights and 'easy grip weights' available. Some of you may find that exercises using resistance bands (wide elastic bands, as shown in Chapter 12) will be best because of grip strength problems. These can provide just as good a workout as weights.

THE BOTTOM LINE

It doesn't matter whether you are over 40 or over 80, or whether you have some form of arthritis, the principles of training remain the same.

Chapter 3

Overweight or 'fat'— what does it really mean?

> *'Facts do not cease
> to exist because they
> are ignored.'*
>
> ALDOUS HUXLEY

When we think of someone as being fat or overweight we do so without first checking on their age, weight and height, or consulting a chart. It's just something we recognise. There's stuff bulging out in the wrong places. In men it's usually a stomach that bulges way over the belt, and in women, well, they're sort of wider than they should be—especially over the hips—and there are extra bits at the back of their upper arms where the triceps should be. Yet there are men and women we don't think of as being overweight or fat but who weigh just as much as those people who to us look 'fat'. What's going on? Why do some people look fat and others not, even though they're of similar height and weight? What's going on is that those people who don't appear fat are not bulging in the wrong places.

Remember the primary school riddle? Which weighs more, a kilo of rocks or a kilo of feathers? They may weigh the same but they certainly look different, just as a kilo of fat looks very different from a kilo of muscle—and importantly it occupies a much larger space. Fatty tissue bulges, flops and jiggles—what's more it does so even in people who appear to be underweight! Touch it and it feels exactly the same in both fat and thin people. How can underweight people still have fat? I'll tell you that too, shortly.

Muscle is different from fat. It certainly feels different—it's firm and it doesn't flop about. Sure, if there's a lot of it about it 'bulges' but when you look at people with muscles that bulge you don't think of them as being overweight or fat, because bulging muscle is firm and it follows the body's normal shape. Muscle enhances the body's shape rather than altering it in a negative way. In fact it makes people look leaner, which is perhaps why we describe muscle in terms of 'lean body mass'.

WHAT'S WRONG WITH BEING FAT?

If fat is what you want then fat is your right. Life is about choices and as adults we are entitled to make our own decisions. Some overweight people rationalise their condition by making a joke about it, 'I'm fat and I'm happy' or 'Whenever I think about exercise I lie down until the thought goes away'. Maybe there are some people who are truly satisfied with the way things are for them, but I've never met an overweight person who after losing weight in an exercise program said, 'Gee, I hate the new me—I was much happier when I was overweight'.

The problem with being fat is not the way it looks on the outside, although for many this is the prime motivation for wanting to do something about it. The real problem is what is happening on the inside. In the western world obesity is increasingly being recognised as a modern-day health problem. The 1995 Australian National Nutrition Survey found that 56% of adult Australians were overweight or obese, which incidentally makes this potentially the largest illness epidemic ever faced by this country. We are not alone. In January 2001 the United States Surgeon General announced a national action plan in an attempt to reduce the prevalence of overweight and obesity.

NASTY FAT FACTS

Being overweight is a known risk factor for a number of conditions.

1. HEART (CARDIOVASCULAR) DISEASE

This occurs because fatty plaques, made up of cholesterol and other fats, form in the blood vessels of the heart known as the coronary arteries. As you know, blood carries oxygen to our muscles and to other tissues. When we exercise, our muscles require more oxygen to cope with the extra work we're asking them to do. The heart has to pump faster to provide this. Because the heart is beating (pumping) faster, the heart muscle itself requires more oxygen. This oxygen is delivered to the heart muscle via the coronary arteries. However, if the coronary arteries are narrowed by fatty plaques, not enough blood and oxygen reaches the heart muscle to cope with the extra work it has to do while pumping faster. This lack of oxygen to the heart muscle causes pain (known as angina), which is usually felt in the centre of the chest. If the heart muscle is deprived of oxygen for too long then part of the muscle will actually die, and this is what is referred to as a 'heart attack' (or myocardial infarction). Of course, if too much of the heart muscle dies, the heart will fail to pump altogether and then we won't have to worry about diet, fat, exercise—or anything else.

In some people, the coronary arteries are so narrowed by fatty plaques that angina can occur even at rest, particularly if the heart rate increases as a result of anxiety or excitement. This is why in people with severe narrowing of the coronary arteries, heart attacks can be caused simply by the excitement of watching sporting events, let alone participating.

What is of particular concern is that, despite great advances in medical technology and treatment, cardiovascular disease kills more Australians than any other disease—in fact one death every 10 minutes.

2. STROKE

Where blood vessels to the brain are narrowed by fatty plaques, the flow of blood can be so slowed down that a blood clot develops, cutting off blood flow to the brain. A stroke can result, which can leave you permanently disabled by paralysis, blindness, loss of speech or brain damage.

3. DISEASE OF THE LEG ARTERIES

Where blood vessels to the leg muscles are narrowed by fatty plaques, the lack of blood flow to these muscles can result in severe pain, usually felt in the calf muscles. This comes on with walking, when the oxygen demands of the leg muscles exceed the blood vessels' capacity to supply them with sufficient blood.

4. HIGH BLOOD PRESSURE

Population studies indicate that 75% of high blood pressure can be directly attributed to obesity. High blood pressure is sometimes referred to as the 'silent killer' (as is osteoporosis) because many people who have it are unaware of it. High blood pressure means that the heart has to work much harder in order to pump out blood against the increased resistance of tight, narrow vessels, and in time this can lead to heart failure, kidney damage and stroke.

5. DIABETES

Being overweight, and in particular having a 'fat stomach' (abdominal obesity), is recognised as a significant risk factor for the onset of diabetes in adults. The reason is simple. High levels of certain dietary fats inside the body's cells make these cells resistant to the effects of insulin. This is referred to as 'insulin resistance', and, since insulin is the body's hormone responsible for getting sugar (in the form of glucose) into cells, the result is a high blood sugar level. This is diabetes. Being obese and diabetic represents a 'double whammy' because, independently of obesity, diabetes is a significant risk factor for heart disease and stroke and can also cause kidney failure and blindness.

6. OSTEOARTHRITIS (DEGENERATIVE JOINT DISEASE)

Being overweight is recognised as the most important contributor to the risk of developing osteoarthritis of the knees, exceeding even the risk imposed by knee injury, knee surgery and family history. It also increases the risk of osteoarthritis of other joints in the legs.

7. CANCER

Being overweight is now a recognised risk factor for certain types of cancer, particularly cancer of the bowel, breast and ovary.

THE FEAR FACTOR

Many people with heart disease, high blood pressure and diabetes—and sometimes even their doctors—are fearful that exercise may be dangerous. However a recent study of more than 2000 people aged 40 years or older with two or more of the following conditions—heart disease, high blood pressure, diabetes or high blood fat levels (cholesterol and/or triglycerides)—found that those who were exercising less than 30 minutes a week were more likely to die within the next 42 months than those who were more active. We now know that older, sicker patients may be the very people who benefit most from exercise. As you read further on in this book you will see how a 'safety first' approach to exercise can minimise the risks and maximise the benefits of exercise.

THE BOTTOM LINE

By avoiding obesity, we can reduce the risk of heart disease, stroke, arterial disease, high blood pressure, diabetes, osteoarthritis and various types of cancer.

4 The metabolism
and
muscle story

> 'Whatever women do they
> must do twice as well as
> men to be thought half
> as good. Luckily this is
> not difficult.'
>
> CHARLOTTE WHITTON

METABOLIC RATE

You often hear overweight people saying 'I just have to look at food
and I put on weight'. Obviously that's not true. It's a metaphor for
saying, 'I seem to eat very little, I never feel satisfied or even full but
I still put on weight'. And that *is* true! How is this possible? Are we
genetically programmed to be fat irrespective of what we do?
Of course there are genetic differences. Some people do have more fat
cells than others and there are individual differences in metabolic
rate—the rate at which our bodies burn energy (kilojoules or
calories). A person with a *higher* metabolic rate will burn *more
kilojoules* and consequently less will be stored as fat. However we
now know that, whatever your genetic 'program', it can be
reprogrammed.

HOW TO CHANGE YOUR METABOLIC RATE FROM
SLOW TO FAST

The first thing to appreciate is that body fat (adipose tissue) is not
metabolically active. Once it's there, it just sits there like a dead
weight (in more ways than one). Of course it's not completely useless
and fat does have some important functions—for example, it

provides a source of reserve energy and is also an insulator against the cold. But the more body fat you've got, the less efficiently you'll burn kilojoules. This partly explains why people who carry lots of body fat also gain weight so easily when they seemingly eat very little. They simply lack the ability to burn kilojoules efficiently. The result—these surplus kilojoules, whether they come from carbohydrate, protein or dietary fat, are stored as body fat, weight increases and the resting metabolic rate falls further. And it gets worse. Because of the excess fat, exercise becomes difficult, you tire easily, you do less, and the result is further weight gain. This is perhaps the most vicious of vicious cycles.

Now muscle, unlike fat, *is* metabolically active. *Even when you are not exercising*, 1 kilogram of muscle is burning 323.4 kilojoules per day just to maintain itself. Compare this to 1 kilogram of fat, which burns only 18.5 kilojoules to maintain itself. And what happens to the unused kilojoules? You guessed it—they're stored as body fat. Pretty staggering numbers, aren't they? Perhaps even food for thought! The more muscle you have, the higher will be your metabolic rate and the more efficiently you'll burn those kilojoules that otherwise would get stored as fat.

Men have an advantage over women because their larger muscle mass means that they have a naturally higher metabolic rate. This is why men can generally eat more than women and not gain as much weight—but not forever. In men and in women the metabolic rate falls as we get older. It's not that our metabolic rate 'ages' as we age. It happens because as we get older we lose muscle mass and gain fat. There are now scientific studies that have demonstrated that it's possible for people even over 70 years of age to restore their declining metabolic rate to what it was in their thirties. This makes it possible to eat more as we get older and, almost unbelievably, not gain weight. Give me the 'magic pill', I hear you say. Sorry, folks, there's no pill—and that's the good news.

Perhaps you're also thinking that the solution is obvious: 'I'll get rid of body fat by dieting and then build up some muscles so that I can increase my metabolic rate—end of problem'. I imagine that literally millions of people have gone down this path—and failed. Why won't it work? After all, it sounds quite logical.

WHY DOESN'T DIETING WORK FOREVER?

Dieting won't work because when you go on a weight reduction diet, particularly of the 'crash' variety, the first thing you will lose is fluid. Next you *lose muscle* and, significantly (and perhaps less well known), you also lose bone. You lose what we call lean tissue or lean body mass. Now all those kilojoules that were previously being used up to maintain muscle metabolism will be stored as body fat. The more radical the diet the more lean tissue is lost. Eventually you'll also lose body fat but by then you've lost so much muscle you are tired, weak and have no energy. You're also depressed because you are depriving yourself of one of life's essentials and pleasures— food. In fact, you feel so tired and miserable that exercise is the very last thing on your mind. What's more, without your knowing it, your body's survival mechanisms have come into play, resulting in your metabolic rate falling even further so as to better conserve the few kilojoules you are taking in.

Your scales will tell you that you've lost weight, but what they won't tell you is that one-third of this is from a loss of muscle, bone and other lean tissue. The result—you cannot function efficiently at home or at work, and all of the evidence shows that no-one can deprive themselves indefinitely. When, inevitably, your tortured body and your willpower cave in and you start eating again, your by-now depressed metabolic rate will ensure that you're an even more efficient fat-storing machine! Furthermore you've lost so much muscle by dieting it's going to be even more difficult to exercise sufficiently to accomplish anything. What you've just succeeded in doing is trading one vicious cycle for another.

Remember I said you can be underweight and still be 'fat'? If you happen to know someone who has done the diet-torture routine, ask if he or she would mind if you felt their 'muscles'. Feel their upper arms and calf muscles. You're in for a shock. What you'll feel is soft, floppy toneless tissue on a thin body. What you're feeling is fat on a body that's lost muscle. It's all pretty horrible, but thankfully easily avoided. By now I hope this reality is dawning: dieting does not achieve lasting or worthwhile weight loss, nor will it make any difference to your cardiovascular fitness. On the other hand, exercise-induced weight loss *will* reduce total body fat *and* significantly improve cardiovascular fitness.

MUSCLE

Muscle supports our skeleton and gives our body stability. Without functioning muscle we couldn't move, breathe, eat or even swallow. People with wasting diseases of muscle or diseases that paralyse the nerves that cause muscle to move lose these functions and cannot survive. In older adults who don't have muscle or nerve disease but who haven't taken steps to preserve their muscle strength, muscle weakness can also lead to death. Because muscles support and stabilise the skeleton, having weak muscles means a loss of stability, which increases the risk of a fall—and when older people fall they break bones, especially hips. This is a significant cause of death in the older age groups.

HOW TO STOP THE DECLINE—THE GOOD NEWS

It has been estimated that women lose about 2 kilograms of muscle mass every 10 years after the age of 30—and the process accelerates after the menopause. In men the same process occurs but begins slightly later. This is associated with reduced strength, bone loss, a lower metabolic rate, increased body fat and changes in body shape. A number of studies have now shown that resistance training can produce muscle gains for older people in as little as eight weeks. Furthermore it has been shown that 12 months of resistance training will not only arrest the loss of muscle mass associated with ageing, but will significantly increase it—without having to resort to drugs such as steroids, human growth hormone or stimulants. Even during the first few years after the menopause, when the rate of muscle and bone loss is greatest, resistance training has been shown to significantly increase lean body mass (muscle and bone) and strength.

A recent collaborative study involving investigators in America and Australia has provided us with the first convincing evidence that, even in the very elderly in whom muscle mass has been lost because of increasing age, underuse and undernutrition, resistance training coupled with adequate nutrition can actually reverse age-related muscle changes and restore muscle mass. This is accompanied by a huge increase in strength. The investigators pointed out that it's only training that requires high force muscle contractions—which is what resistance training does—that can achieve these outcomes. It can be achieved by lifting free weights (weight training using barbells, dumb-bells, etc.), by using 'resistance equipment' (weight machines), by lifting your own weight (push-ups, chin-ups, sit-ups, dips) and by resistance band (wide elastic band) exercise.

Importantly these investigators also found that in resistance training it was not just the 'concentric' contractions that were important in building muscle but also the 'eccentric' contractions. Concentric contractions describe the lifting or 'power' phase of weight training while eccentric contractions describe the lowering or 'relaxation' phase. In fact, to everyone's surprise, it was found that it was the lowering rather than the lifting of weights which was more important in strength building. We will return to this point later on in the book when we discuss exercise technique. It's extremely important, and I don't mind admitting it's a pet theme of mine.

HOW DO MUSCLES GET BIGGER AND STRONGER?

If you wished to only develop muscle strength then you would use heavy weights (requiring near maximum effort) and do no more than six repetitions per set (see Chapter 12). If on the other hand you were using weights to try to develop endurance then you'd use light weights with a large number of repetitions (20 or more). The resistance training programs described in this book are designed to simultaneously build muscle strength and endurance, which is why I generally advise 8–12 repetitions per set. Remember that any magnitude of overload will build muscle and strength but heavier weights (near your maximum) will result in a greater training effect.

It's known that gains in muscle mass and muscle strength occur through a process of 'microdamage' to muscle fibres, a natural process of breaking down and re-forming of small muscle elements. The collaborative study referred to earlier showed for the first time that resistance training in humans resulted in the reappearance of muscle elements which are normally seen only during early development. This regeneration process occurred in muscle fibres that had been severely atrophied (shrivelled) through age, underuse and poor nutrition. The investigators confirmed that the stimulus for muscle regeneration and muscle building was microdamage, which could only be achieved using what's called the 'progressive muscle overload principle' through resistance training. Their final conclusion was that age-related muscle loss can be modified even in individuals as old as 98 years of age.

THE BOTTOM LINE

You can only maintain weight loss by eating and by exercising.

Chapter 5 Food and diet

> *'The years that a woman subtracts from her age are not lost. They are added to the ages of other women.'*
>
> DIANE DE POITIERS

It is impossible to avoid a discussion on diet and nutrition when considering a physical training program. I don't want you to give up what you consider to be the 'good things in life', unless of course they happen to be especially bad for you—for some people the 'good things in life' are not necessarily 'good for life'. However at the end of the day you will make your own decisions. The purpose of this chapter is to give you the information so that you are in a position to make informed decisions and choices.

Knowing what is good, not so good and just plain bad in your diet can be helpful. It may enable you to adjust the goalposts rather than move them altogether. We are talking about a permanent adjustment that will enhance your life and provide permanent results, not a temporary 'quick fix' that you'll be inclined to abandon because it's impractical or too radical. There would be absolutely no point in improving your strength and cardiovascular fitness through training if your diet made you miserable. After all, the whole point of exercise is to enhance your enjoyment of life. Food and alcohol are part of that enjoyment. If you decide to accept the challenge of my resistance training and cardiovascular training programs you won't need to eat less—only less of the wrong stuff. It is never necessary to feel hungry. In fact, many of you are likely to be eating more than you ever did before.

We'll identify the foods that are obviously bad for you. In giving these things up you shouldn't see yourself as having made a sacrifice. In fact what you have done is *stopped* making a sacrifice— of yourself.

THE FOOD TYPES

Broadly speaking, the foods that are bad for you are those that are high in kilojoules and low in nutritional value (e.g. sugar, syrup, sweets and pastries) and of course our old foe 'bad fats', which we'll discuss in Chapter 6. I don't advise obsessive calorie counting but you may find it helpful to keep these numbers in mind:

- 1 gram of fat contains 37 kilojoules (9 calories)
- 1 gram of carbohydrate contains 16 kilojoules (4 calories)
- 1 gram of protein contains 17 kilojoules (4 calories).

(And for your information, 1 gram of alcohol contains 29 kilojoules (7 calories).)

Surplus kilojoules from any food source will be converted to body fat, but remember that dietary fat contains more kilojoules per gram than other foods and is converted into body fat with little metabolic effort (i.e. it requires fewer kilojoules to complete the process than does metabolising carbohydrate and protein). It's also harder for the body to access the kilojoules from body fat than from carbohydrate.

Let's now look a bit more closely at the three food types: carbohydrate, protein and fat.

CARBOHYDRATE

Carbohydrate consists of unrefined carbohydrate and sugars. Unrefined carbohydrate, once known as 'complex carbohydrate', should constitute most of your carbohydrate intake—all vegetables, fruit, legumes (peas, beans), pasta, rice, cereal grains (as found in unsugared breakfast cereal), oats and wholemeal bread. Many of these unrefined carbohydrates also contain important vitamins, trace minerals, dietary fibre and other protective components. Dietary fibre is vitally important because it helps to remove cholesterol from the body (more on cholesterol in Chapter 6), reduces the risk of bowel cancer, prevents or reduces the symptoms of irritable bowel syndrome, and prevents constipation.

The healthiest forms of sugar are those found in fruit—all fruit—and in milk. The amount of kilojoules in fruit is modest (even a large portion of fruit won't deliver more than about 600 kilojoules), and fruit is a valuable source of vitamins, minerals, dietary fibre and antioxidants (see later in this chapter). If you make the effort to eliminate from your diet high-kilojoule, low-nutritional-value sugars (sweets, pastries, biscuits, cakes and carbonated soft drinks), you will from time to time experience a craving for something sweet. This is where fruit comes to the rescue with low-kilojoule 'good' sugars and all the other valuable goodies you won't find in pastries, biscuits, cakes etc.

PROTEIN

Protein is found in fish, meat, poultry, eggs, dairy products, nuts and tofu (soybean curd). The amount of protein found in meat pies and sausages continues to be a matter of contemporary debate in Australia. In any event, the high fat content of these products means they should be eaten only infrequently—once every three or four years would be about right!

Recently there's been a revival of interest in high-protein, high-fat, low-carbohydrate diets which were once popular in the 1970s. The diet allows unlimited meat and fat and bans unrefined carbohydrate (potatoes, rice, pasta, grains, legumes, fruit and most vegetables). Its rationale is that, despite people eating less fat, obesity is on the increase so that dietary fat can't be the culprit. This is a fallacy. In fact most studies show that people are not eating less fat, they are just unaware of the number of foods containing fat, such as full-cream dairy products, cheese, chips, biscuits, pastries and snack foods.

When carbohydrate intake is restricted the body converts dietary protein and bodily protein (lean muscle tissue) to glucose.

The products of this protein breakdown are then excreted through the kidneys, and this has been shown to cause kidney damage. Other dangers of the diet include an increased risk of heart disease (because the high fat in the diet raises blood fat levels), vitamin deficiency, fatigue, weakness (because of a loss of lean muscle tissue) and potentially an increased cancer risk because of a low fruit intake. High-protein, high-fat, low carbohydrate diets are not recommended.

We require protein for muscle and bone growth because it contains the nine essential amino acids which can only be obtained from food (they are called 'essential' because our bodies cannot manufacture them). However studies have failed to show convincing evidence that muscle building can be accelerated by diets that are very high in protein and contain little carbohydrate and fat, particularly when compared to the more balanced diet I am proposing.

Remember the kilojoule figures for fat, carbohydrate and protein mentioned earlier? Protein is low in kilojoules, but protein-containing foods also come with fat, especially dairy products (with the exception of skim milk). Logic therefore dictates that we choose protein with the following characteristics: (1) low fat and (2) 'good fat'. This means fish, lean meat (with the visible fat cut off), low-fat dairy products (especially low-fat cottage cheese) and tofu. If you're a nut freak, almonds and walnuts, which are very low in 'bad' (saturated) fat and moderately high in 'good' (unsaturated) fat, are also good. In fact, in general all nuts are good. Incidentally, if you're a 'snacker', almonds (or olives) are great—forget the chips and biscuits.

There are now sound scientific reasons for relying on fish and other marine life as your main source of protein, chief of which are the special properties in the polyunsaturated fats that are to be found in fish. And because fish has less fat than meat it also has fewer kilojoules. More on this shortly. Vegetarians need an alternative source of protein but can take heart from some recently published research indicating that 25–50 grams of soy protein a day will significantly reduce levels of LDL (low-density lipoprotein) cholesterol (so-called 'bad' cholesterol). In fact the American Heart Association suggests that even non-vegetarians with high blood cholesterol levels would benefit from substituting soy for animal protein. Vegetarians can obtain all the essential amino acids from a balanced diet that includes soy, green leafy vegetables, eggs, dairy products, beans, rice, corn, nuts, buckwheat, lentils, pumpkin seeds and sunflower seeds.

FATS

An understanding of the health effects of the different types of dietary fat is important in being able to make informed decisions on how we should deal with fat in our diet. For this reason Chapter 6 will deal exclusively with this topic.

OTHER FACTS ABOUT DIET
WATER

I very much doubt that anyone reading this book drinks enough water. If you are exercising, your water intake becomes critical. It's important not only to replace the water you lose through sweating and breathing but in the course of exercising it is vital to have sufficient water to help mobilise your energy stores. You can be reasonably sure that if you are having a bad training session and feel particularly flat it's probably because you haven't drunk enough water. You can confirm this by checking the colour of your urine—if it's yellow you're dehydrated. We're talking a minimum of 8 standard glasses of water a day.

SALT

In the recent past it was advised that people who were exercising regularly take extra salt. Now we know this is not necessary. The more salt you have the more salt you will *lose* in your sweat and the more dehydrated you are likely to become. People with high blood pressure in particular should avoid a high salt intake and at the same time ensure an adequate intake of fruit, vegetables and low-fat dairy products (which are rich in potassium, calcium, magnesium and protein, and low in saturated fat and cholesterol).

How much salt is too much? For people who don't have high blood pressure, no greater than the equivalent of three teaspoons a day (roughly 5.8 grams of salt) is recommended. For people with high blood pressure, no greater than the equivalent of two teaspoons a day is recommended. Remember that salt is present in cereals, bread, cheese, canned products, processed foods, take-away foods and dairy products.

ALCOHOL

Personally speaking, I love my wine and wouldn't be without it. I imagine that there is almost no red wine drinker alive today who hasn't heard or read that, in moderation, red wine reduces the risk of heart disease. Actually white wine does the same thing. It appears to do so by increasing HDL ('good') cholesterol levels but it is only red wine that makes blood less 'sticky' and thereby reduces the risk of thrombosis (blood clot formation). There is however a 'but'—isn't there always? Alcohol is high in kilojoules and too much of it will increase the level of another body fat, triglycerides, which can contribute to heart disease—yet another example of 'too much of a good thing'. Even for those of you who exercise up to 4 or 5 times a week, it's recommended that you drink in moderation and have one or two alcohol-free days a week.

TOBACCO

If you're a smoker then you cannot expect to reduce your biological age by training and by good diet. While he was dying from lung cancer Yul Brynner said, 'For God's sake, DON'T SMOKE'. My uncle Sonny—ex-prisoner of war, lifesaver, boxer, horserider, motor rally champ and actor—a strong man, is dying from lung disease caused by cigarette smoking. Death by 1000 cuts. He told me, 'If you know anyone who smokes tell them about your uncle Sonny.' So now I'm telling you.

ANTIOXIDANTS AND FREE RADICALS

Unlike the name suggests, free radicals are not necessarily unrestrained political activists. They are a by-product of the metabolism of our body's cells. We all have free radicals. They are unstable molecules that are thought to play a role in cell ageing (and hence the ageing process). Fortunately the body also has other molecules, known as antioxidants, that have the ability to 'mop up' these free radicals. There are many antioxidant compounds contained in food and some of them are vitamins for example, A, C, E and ß-carotene which are found in—fruit (yellow, red and orange), vegetables, soy/tofu, garlic, leeks, onions, red wine, tea, nuts and oils. Studies have found that a moderate to high intake of these antioxidants reduces the risk of heart disease, Alzheimer's disease, stroke, bowel cancer and breast cancer. A large Swedish study found that a low intake of fruit and vegetables significantly increased the risk of bowel cancer especially involving the rectum. Of particular interest is that the antioxidant vitamins A, C and E protect against breast cancer, but only where these vitamins are consumed as food and not taken as supplements. Similar data exist with respect to dietary vitamin E protecting against heart disease, provided it is consumed as food and not as a supplement. In older people, vitamin C might help protect against degenerative diseases of the eyes such as cataracts and macular degeneration.

VITAMINS AND MINERALS

I cannot overemphasise the importance of eating adequate amounts of fruit and vegetables. I suspect that because there's so much of it about and it is relatively inexpensive, familiarity and affordability have bred contempt. Perhaps if they were more of a 'luxury' people might eat more of them. Many people appear to have turned their back on fruit in favour of confectionery—sweets and biscuits. Yet fruit and vegetables are our source of a wide range of vitamins—not only antioxidant vitamins but importantly the large B group of vitamins—as well as being a source of minerals and dietary fibre. It's from vegetables that we largely get folic acid (a B group vitamin), which among its other benefits may also protect against heart disease and bowel cancer.

Fruit, vegetables and low-fat dairy products are a source of potassium and magnesium, minerals which reduce the risk of high blood pressure and stroke, see the section on salt in this chapter. Eat fruit and vegetables and save money on expensive vitamin supplements.

Zinc is a mineral which is important in helping to maintain immune function. A deficiency may be associated with chest and gastric infections. However high-dose zinc supplementation may suppress immune function and increase the risk of heart disease (by increasing LDL cholesterol levels). Zinc should therefore be consumed only in its natural form in oysters, lean lamb and beef, fortified breakfast cereals and baked beans.

Contemporary medical studies suggest that as we get older, we need more calcium in our diets. Calcium is important to maintain the strength of our bones. This is particularly true for women, who start off with a smaller bone mass than men. After the menopause, women lose bone quite rapidly as a result of significant falls in circulating oestrogen levels. Calcium supplements do slow bone loss in post menopausal women but may still fail to reduce the risk of fracture. You should consult your doctor to see whether you are at risk of osteoporosis and whether hormone replacement therapy or medications are required in addition to calcium supplementation. Women over 40 should have three to four serves of low-fat dairy food daily. What we do know is that the best type of exercise to prevent osteoporosis is resistance exercise, or, alternatively, high impact aerobics. What these two types of exercise have in common is that they both place a significant load on the bone, which helps to increase bone density and to reduce bone loss.

FIBRE FACTS

I know—mention dietary fibre and you think 'he's telling us about fibre because he thinks we're old and constipated'. Hey—I'm talking to me too! That's not why I think it's worth talking about dietary fibre. I know that if you follow my training programs and keep up your water intake you won't be constipated. I'm telling you about fibre because there may be some stuff you don't know about. Here are some fibre facts.

- A fibre-rich diet lowers blood cholesterol.
- A fibre-rich diet lowers blood pressure.
- A fibre-rich diet can substantially reduce the risk of coronary heart disease and heart attack.
- A fibre-rich diet reduces the risk of bowel cancer, breast cancer and irritable bowel syndrome.

Welcome to 'fibre-space'. Seek and consume oats, oat bran, cereal grains, wholegrain bread, fruit, vegetables, barley, legumes and fresh ground linseed (which also has the advantage of containing Omega 3 fats, see Chapter 6).

THE 'EAT HEALTHY NEVER FEEL HUNGRY' PRINCIPLE

I have intentionally not 'prescribed' a specific diet in this book. As I said at the beginning of this chapter, it was my wish only to provide the information so you can decide for yourself. I am quite certain that the last thing the world needs is yet another diet, let alone one from a non-dietician. However I suspect that if you've decided to follow my training programs you won't want to sabotage your own hard-earned training gains by eating badly. On this basis I suggest you follow this basic principle: EAT HEALTHY AND NEVER FEEL HUNGRY.

Think of yourself as a bomb disposal expert. By excluding from your diet foods that have poor nutritional value, are very high in kilojoules or which are known to increase the risk of cardiovascular disease, you have just begun the delicate process of defusing a time bomb. You may not be able to stop the fuse from burning but you can make it burn a whole lot slower.

You probably thought that Egypt was the home of the pyramids. Maybe, but everyone it seems is getting into the act. We have the

United States Department of Agriculture Food Guide Pyramid, the Healthy Diet Pyramid of the Australian Nutrition Foundation, the Cholesterol Control Pyramid, etc. Relax, because here is my food pyramid with apologies to the Egyptians and other pyramid makers. This pyramid is called the 'Live Stronger—Live Longer Pyramid'.

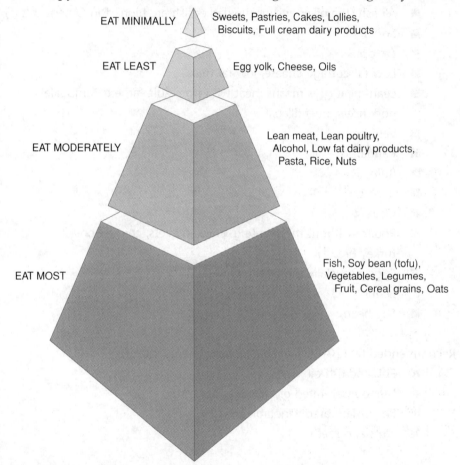

EAT MINIMALLY — Sweets, Pastries, Cakes, Lollies, Biscuits, Full cream dairy products

EAT LEAST — Egg yolk, Cheese, Oils

EAT MODERATELY — Lean meat, Lean poultry, Alcohol, Low fat dairy products, Pasta, Rice, Nuts

EAT MOST — Fish, Soy bean (tofu), Vegetables, Legumes, Fruit, Cereal grains, Oats

Recommended unrefined (or minimally refined) carbohydrate (50–60% of total dietary energy intake)

- Rice (brown better than white and only steamed)
- All pasta
- All vegetables
- Legumes (peas, beans)
- All fruit

- Cereal grains, wholemeal bread, oats
- Non-fat yoghurt (not frozen yoghurt)
- Low-fat milk products

Recommended protein (20–30% of total dietary energy intake)
- All fish (the oilier and/or the darker fish are highest in Omega 3 fats)
- Squid
- Octopus
- Low-fat cottage cheese, low-fat milk
- Lean meat (this means meat with no visible fat, e.g. lamb fillets, pork fillets, beef fillets)
- Venison
- Kangaroo
- Buffalo
- Rabbit
- Goat
- Poultry without the skin (e.g. chicken fillets, chicken breast, turkey breast)
- Eggs, especially those with Omega 3
- Lentils
- Soy bean

Recommended fat (20–30% of total dietary energy intake)
- Fish and fish oil
- Monounsaturated oils (canola, olive, soy)
- Polyunsaturated vegetable oils
- Nuts and seeds

THE BOTTOM LINE

Weight loss is important only if you're overweight—don't be obsessed with weight loss. Focus on becoming fitter and stronger by following my exercise programs and weight loss will happen as a by-product of your training.

Chapter 6

The fat
story

| *'There is dignity in
personal appearance.'*
YAMAMOTO TSUNETOMO,
THE BOOK OF THE SAMURAI (HAGAKURE)

This is an important story. I urge you to read it carefully—and then read it again. This background knowledge may help you in your quest to change. It may even 'save' or at least prolong your life. If you know how something works it's that much easier to understand why it might be good or bad for you.

Fat and oil are one and the same thing. It's just that one is solid and the other liquid. So-called 'saturated' fats—found in fatty meat, poultry, lard, pork dripping, full cream dairy products, palm oil and coconut oil—are solid at room temperature. The 'unsaturated' fats— found in fish, fish oil, vegetable oils, nuts, seeds and avocado—are liquid at room temperature. When we talk of saturated or unsaturated fats in our food, we are saying that *most* of the fat in a particular food is saturated or unsaturated. There is almost always a mixture of different fats in food.

SATURATED FATS AND CHOLESTEROL
The problem with a diet high in saturated fats—full-cream dairy products, cheese, shortbread, cheesecake, pastries, lamb chops, salami—is that these fats raise blood levels of LDL ('bad') cholesterol. LDL cholesterol is 'bad' because it transports cholesterol into the arteries of the body, unlike HDL (high-density lipoprotein) cholesterol or 'good' cholesterol, which transports cholesterol out of the vessels. Remember it is cholesterol that forms part of those nasty,

fatty plaques that narrow our arteries. Saturated fats increase LDL cholesterol levels by interfering with our body's ability to get rid of excess cholesterol. People often mistakenly focus purely on the cholesterol content of foods but, except for a few foods like egg yolks, caviar and offal (brains, kidneys, liver, sweet breads) which are extremely high in cholesterol, *it is generally the saturated fat content of food that is the problem*. In fact, compared to dietary saturated fat, cholesterol in food has a much less significant effect in raising blood LDL cholesterol levels.

When you buy a packet of chips or pretzels that states 'cholesterol free' this is not telling you that the product is 'fat free', nor even that it is free of saturated fat! 'Cholesterol free' foods are frequently cooked in palm oil, which is a saturated fat. Not only will you still get a hefty dose of kilojoules, *but the saturated fat will raise LDL cholesterol levels even though there is no cholesterol in the food itself*. Where a product is labelled 'non-fat' or 'fat-free', read the product information carefully—some of these products are still high in kilojoules because simple sugars and refined carbohydrates have been substituted for fats.

UNSATURATED FATS

Unsaturated fats in our food may be mostly polyunsaturated—such as in fish, fish oil, lentils, kidney beans and various vegetable oils (sunflower, safflower, soy and corn)—or mostly monounsaturated, as in avocados, olive oil and canola oil. There two kinds of polyunsaturated fat, Omega 3 and Omega 6. Omega 3 fats predominate in fish and fish oil and are present in smaller amounts in canola oil, soybean oil and linseed. Omega 6 fats predominate in most vegetable oils. In fact vegetable oils and margarine are our chief dietary source of polyunsaturated fats. These polyunsaturated fats (Omega 3 and Omega 6) have cholesterol-lowering effects, which is why I recommend them. But remember this: *the cholesterol-elevating effects of saturated fats are twice as potent as the cholesterol-lowering effects of unsaturated fats*, which is why I recommend that you keep your saturated fat intake to an absolute minimum. I should also add that, if you have arthritis (in particular rheumatoid arthritis) or certain inflammatory disorders such as psoriasis, Omega 3 fats are preferable to Omega 6 fats (see later in this chapter).

TRANS-FATTY ACIDS

You don't hear much about trans-fatty acids but they are important —for all the wrong reasons. Not only do they raise blood levels of 'bad' (LDL) cholesterol and lower the levels of 'good' (HDL) cholesterol, a recent study found that they increase the risk of adult-onset (type II) diabetes. Trans-fatty acids are found in margarines, biscuits and many snack foods.

'OILS AIN'T OILS'

Remember that popular TV ad 'Oils ain't oils'? Well, it's certainly true of oils (fats) in our diet. Because of the well-publicised dangers of saturated fats many health-conscious people, irrespective of their exercise habits, have switched from saturated fats to unsaturated fats for everyday cooking. However, even health-conscious people not infrequently buy pre-prepared supermarket dishes, take-aways or fast food with little idea of their fat content. Did you know that one-third of all the money spent on food in Australia is on foods prepared and eaten outside of the family home? It's a similar story in other western countries. The problem is that food prepared outside of our homes often contains much more fat than home-prepared meals.

The fast food industry exists because it fulfils a need. Modern life is fast and we've demanded and have been given a quick food fix. People vaguely understand that this food may be high in fat but may fail to appreciate that it's not the same sort of fat they're using in their own kitchens. Up until only recently most people have had little idea of the fat content of much of the processed and packaged foods that we consume. Luckily this will soon change in Australia with new food labelling laws that require content information on saturated fats, carbohydrate, sugars and protein. For example, many people may be unaware that popular biscuits, snack foods and pastries are often made with palm oil and coconut oil, which contain a higher percentage of saturated fat than any other food—including full-cream dairy products and animal fat! Products cooked in palm oil or coconut oil are therefore just as potentially bad for us as foods cooked in animal-derived saturated fats such as lard (rendered pig fat) and tallow (beef fat), which are commonly used in fast food and take-aways and which won't be affected by the new food labelling laws.

Speak to a take-away food proprieter. He'll tell you he uses 'solid fry' (essentially lard) for all of his cooking. And why does he do this? Simple—it makes everything he cooks crispier and crunchier. If he used what we would consider to be very much healthier polyunsaturated or monounsaturated oil he'd lose 'crispy and crunchy'—and most of his customers. Of course it also means that the cholesterol-lowering effects of the polyunsaturated fats found in fish will be more than wiped out by the cholesterol-elevating effects of the lard in which the fish is fried.

It's 2001—the scientists have done their job—the information is out there—and yet our western diet is still too high in saturated fat. Did you know that currently in Australia one-third of total energy is provided by dietary fat and more than one third of this is from saturated fat? Most of this dietary saturated fat is from dairy products with—believe it or not—biscuits and pastry products contributing as much saturated fat in our diet as meat and poultry. Why is this such a big deal? It's a big deal because an excess of dietary saturated fat is a cause of obesity and cardiovascular disease.

THE FISH STORY

The polyunsaturated fats found in fish are very important because they contain high levels of something very special. This 'something special' is Omega 3 fats. They are special because of their extraordinary health benefits. We now have extensive scientific evidence showing that in communities in which there is a high dietary intake of Omega 3 fats there is a much lower incidence of cardiovascular disease, cardiovascular death, stroke, rheumatoid arthritis and diseases involving inflammation, such as psoriasis and asthma. If this is not a terrific reason to rely on fish (and other marine life) as our predominant source of protein I don't know what is, presuming of course that you're not a vegetarian.

Unlike fish, which contains predominantly Omega 3 fats, meat and poultry are low in Omega 3 fats and significantly higher in saturated fats, while the polyunsaturated vegetable oils contain abundant amounts of Omega 6 fats. Interestingly, gamey meat such as kangaroo is reasonably rich in Omega 3 fats. The traditional western diet, which tends to rely more on meat and poultry than fish for its protein source, and makes use of polyunsaturated vegetable oils, thus leads to a higher Omega 6 intake.

OMEGA 3 VS OMEGA 6—WHAT'S THE DIFFERENCE?
Dietary fats are not simply converted into body fat to provide a reserve energy source. They are also incorporated into certain body tissues. In a traditional western diet in which Omega 6 fats predominate, more of this will find its way into body tissues than Omega 3 fats. This is important because Omega 6 fats form the basis of chemical messengers responsible for inflammation in rheumatoid arthritis, osteoarthritis and other conditions. This seems to be at least part of the reason why these conditions are more common and more severe in communities in which dietary Omega 6 fats predominate. On the other hand, scientific studies have shown that dietary Omega 3 fats can suppress the production of these chemical messengers of inflammation, which is why in communities in which dietary Omega 3 fats predominate over Omega 6 fats many of these diseases are either unknown or at least less common or severe.

FOR PEOPLE WITH ARTHRITIS
We now know from recent studies that dietary Omega 3 fats will be better used and will achieve higher tissue levels in the body if the overall intake of Omega 6 fats is low (less than 10 grams a day). This can be achieved by reducing our consumption of fatty foods,

substituting monounsaturated cooking oils such as olive oil and canola oil (which also contains Omega 3) for polyunsaturated vegetable oils, eating three fish meals a week and, for people with arthritis, supplementing the diet with fish oil.

From clinical studies we are now in a position to state that, in the case of rheumatoid arthritis, the evidence of the beneficial effects of Omega 3 fats has achieved the highest standards of scientific proof. Laboratory studies suggest the same may be true in osteoarthritis (degenerative joint disease). In studies of joint inflammation, patient groups showing benefit have generally been given 3 grams a day of the Omega 3 fats to be found in fish—with no adverse health effects. An average adult portion of fish will contain around 1.2 grams of Omega 3 fats. How big is a 'portion'? Make a fist—that's a portion. So try two portions.

All fish is good but the oilier and/or darker fish (such as groper, blue grenadier, swordfish, snook, salmon, red snapper, tommy ruffs, garfish, sardines, herring, mackerel, tuna, flounder, flathead, haddock) will have higher levels of Omega 3 fats. Also high in Omega 3 fats are squid, octopus and all shellfish (scallop, prawn/shrimp, lobster). Although shellfish (and prawns particularly) contain more cholesterol than fish, they have a lower saturated fat content than meat (and fewer kilojoules) and are considered excellent sources of Omega 3 fats.

It is possible to supplement the diet with fish oil capsules. However, a typical 1 gram soft gelatin capsule of fish oil contains no more than 300 milligrams of Omega 3 fats, so this would mean swallowing 10 capsules per day (or more depending on the Omega 3 content), which most people would find awkward, not to mention costly (it works out at between $4 and $5 a day) and a lot less fun than eating fish or shellfish. An alternative is to take 10–20 millilitres of cod liver oil daily (no more). The Omega 3 fat content of this volume of cod liver oil is equivalent to between 10 and 20 of the 1 gram fish capsules. It's also a lot cheaper, costing roughly 20c a day. Note that people who are allergic to fish may react to fish oil due to trace amounts of fish protein in the oil.

My good pal Les Cleland, who has extensively studied the effects of dietary Omega 3 fats, recommends the 'two glass technique' be used to take cod liver oil. The first glass needs to be small enough to put well into the mouth, and a turned out lip to the glass is an advantage. Pour 20–30 millilitres of fruit or vegetable juice (e.g. tomato juice) into the glass, followed by 10–20 millilitres of fish oil. The oil forms a layer on the surface and should not be stirred. Fill the second, standard-sized glass with juice alone. Pick up the first glass with the juice and oil, place it well into the mouth, then pour it to the back of the mouth and swallow in one action (because fish oil is tasted in the front of the mouth this technique will minimise the taste experience). Follow this immediately with the juice from the second glass, which should be drunk slowly (and may be moved about the mouth before swallowing to wash away any oil that may cause an aftertaste). Done correctly, one should experience no fish taste at all. By taking fish oil in this way just before a solid meal and without any further fluids, repeating of the fish taste is minimised. Of course on the days when you're having your fish meal there's no need to have cod liver oil.

FOR PEOPLE WITH (OR AT RISK OF) HEART DISEASE

In people with known cardiovascular (heart) disease or a history of it, a diet high in Omega 3 fats has been shown to have preventative value in coronary artery disease and to reduce the death rate by 50%, and recent studies have shown a significant reduction in the incidence of stroke. Omega 3 fats lower blood levels of 'bad' (LDL) cholesterol, as well as triglyceride levels (see Chapter 5), make blood less 'sticky' (and therefore less likely to form a clot or thrombosis) and, uniquely, reduce the risk of abnormal heart rhythms and sudden death by stabilising heart muscle. In people with high blood pressure Omega 3 fats have been shown to lower blood pressure.

To achieve these cardiovascular benefits does not require the same high level of Omega 3 fats as is required to benefit patients with arthritis. Two to three fish meals a week will suffice without the need for additional fish oil supplementation. An alternative for people who don't like fish is to take 2–3 millilitres of fish oil daily. Remember that for people with heart disease it is especially important to avoid saturated fats. This should be replaced with Omega 3 or Omega 6 polyunsaturates or with monounsaturates to achieve a cholesterol-lowering effect.

FOR PEOPLE WITH (OR AT RISK OF) BOWEL DISEASE

There is evidence that Omega 3 fats may lower the risk of large bowel cancer, and because of their anti-inflammatory effects they may be helpful in managing inflammatory diseases of the bowel such as Crohn's disease.

FOR MEN

A recently published 30-year study found that men who didn't eat fish had a two to three times greater risk of developing prostate cancer. Omega 3 fatty acids have been shown to inhibit the growth of prostate cancer cells. The study suggested that eating oily fish such as sardines, salmon, herring and mackerel significantly reduced the risk of prostate cancer.

A SUMMARY OF THE KEY POINTS IN THE FAT STORY

- Unsaturated fats are much healthier than saturated fats.
- Everyone should consciously keep saturated fat intake to an absolute minimum.
- There are two categories of polyunsaturated fats—Omega 3 and Omega 6.
- Omega 3 fats are found in high amounts in fish and fish oil and in lower amounts in soybean oil and canola oil (which is predominantly a monounsaturated fat but which also contains Omega 3 polyunsaturates).
- Omega 6 fats are found in high amounts in polyunsaturated vegetable oils (sunflower, safflower, soy and corn) and in margarine.
- Monounsaturated oils (such as canola and olive oil) and polyunsaturated oils (Omega 3 and Omega 6) lower 'bad' (LDL) cholesterol levels.

■ Because of the established health benefits in people with arthritis (especially rheumatoid arthritis), dietary Omega 3 fats should be preferred to dietary Omega 6 fats.

THE BOTTOM LINE

THE THREE FAT TENETS (WITH APOLOGIES TO JOSÉ)

Whether you're currently healthy, have arthritis or have heart disease, if you decide to follow my training programs (and even if you don't) I have three recommendations regarding fat consumption:

1. No more than 20–25% of your total daily energy intake should be derived from fat.
2. Substitute polyunsaturated and/or monounsaturated fats for saturated fats.
3. When eating meat or poultry remove visible fat and/or skin.

Chapter **7** Arthritis and pain

> '*Remember, we are not our bodies. Instead, we live inside our bodies and can control and move them with our brains. Caring for and attempting to improve our bodies, or earth-suits if you will, is what fitness is all about.*'
>
> EVERETT AABERG,
> RESISTANCE TRAINING INSTRUCTION

This book is not intended to be a self-help guide to diagnosing arthritis. If you have arthritis (and there are roughly 100 different types), then this is something about which you should consult your family doctor and if necessary a specialist. But it does help to understand what type of arthritis you have and how it may affect the function of your joints, and that is what this chapter's about.

ARTHRITIS IN GENERAL

While there is no form of arthritis for which resistance training and cardiovascular training are inappropriate, it may be necessary to introduce some modifications to enable you to accomplish your goals. In people with very severe arthritis that has limited the range of joint movement or significantly reduced grip strength, it may be necessary to follow a permanently modified program. For others, modifications may be required only at times when the arthritis is going through a painful phase and/or when the overall disease has flared up.

Resistance training is as beneficial for people with arthritis as it is for healthy people. This is because pain caused by arthritis means that the joint is used less. Consequently, the muscles that move the joint become weak and wasted. Not only does this make you weaker but it also makes the joint even more unstable than it may be as a result of the damage caused by the arthritis itself—and unstable arthritic joints are much more painful than stable ones. If the range of movement of your joint is limited by arthritis then it won't be possible to exercise the joint through its full range. This doesn't mean you shouldn't exercise, just that you'll have to perform the exercise only through the extent of your particular range of movement. In many cases, as the muscles become stronger the range of joint movement will increase (much to your surprise). Furthermore, as your muscles get stronger you'll find that your joints will become more stable and less painful.

OSTEOARTHRITIS (DEGENERATIVE JOINT DISEASE)
Osteoarthritis is arthritis in which changes occur in the cartilage that covers the ends of the two bones that form a joint. As we discussed earlier, osteoarthritis becomes more common as we get older. It truly is a disease of life. If you are over 40 years old you will have degenerative changes in your joints even though you may be pain-free. Osteoarthritis changes may occur at a younger age for genetic reasons or because the joint has been damaged by past injury or disease.

The result of osteoarthritis is pain and usually limited joint movement. The leg joints are commonly affected because they are subjected to the body's weight. The heavier the body, the heavier the load, and the more susceptible you'll be to osteoarthritis of the leg joints. The most common joint in the leg to be affected is the joint at the base of the big toe. This is because this joint bears more weight per square centimetre of area than any other joint in the body. It can make walking painful but is usually much less of a problem than arthritis of the hip, knee or ankle. In the arm, the joints most commonly affected are those at the base of the thumb and the top of the shoulder, known as the acromioclavicular joint. In fact, degenerative changes in this joint begin in our twenties, although the joint is not always painful. However, it may limit shoulder mobility and thus cause particular problems with certain exercises. For this reason resistance exercises likely to stress these joints can be modified without in any way compromising the benefits of the exercise.

CHRONIC INFLAMMATORY ARTHRITIS

The word 'chronic' means long-lasting. There are many types of chronic inflammatory arthritis but rheumatoid arthritis is the most common and the most potentially devastating because it can involve many joints on both sides of the body. Other common types of chronic inflammatory arthritis include a large group known as the 'spondyloarthropathies', which includes ankylosing spondylitis, psoriatic arthritis, Reiter's disease and reactive arthritis. Many of these chronic inflammatory joint diseases are progressive and require specialist medical treatment, often with combinations of treatments including exercise. People with these disorders are likely to have a reduced exercise tolerance because the arthritis has usually resulted in a sedentary lifestyle. It's therefore all the more important to proceed gradually. Some people with chronic inflammatory arthritis may prefer to exercise in the afternoon because of the common problem of 'morning stiffness'. Some find it useful to have a warm shower before exercising or to warm the joints and surrounding muscles with special pads called hydrocolator pads.

If you have chronic inflammatory arthritis and your disease is in a very active phase (e.g. your joints are warm, swollen and more painful than usual), then you should limit your exercise to those parts in which the joint inflammation is not active. If your flare-up is widespread, involving all four limbs, then you are advised to get over the flare-up before restarting your exercise program. Additional or alternative exercises for people with arthritis are described in Chapter 14.

ANKYLOSING SPONDYLITIS
This is a particular type of chronic inflammatory arthritis that affects mainly the spinal joints and often affects young people. It usually begins in the pelvis (in the sacroiliac joints) and then may progress up the spine. It causes pain and stiffness, both of which will worsen with rest and improve with exercise. Because the inflammation can affect the upper part of the spine, it can limit movement of the chest and this may affect your cardiovascular training.

FIBROMYALGIA SYNDROME
Fibromyalgia is a condition characterised by widespread pain and tenderness. At one time it was thought to be a disorder of soft tissues and was known as 'fibrositis'. Now we know that the disorder is not in the soft tissues but in the pain system itself. Not only does this result in soft tissue pain and tenderness but it also causes irritability of the bowel, bladder and skin, as well as extreme sensitivity to bright lights and loud noise. We also know two other important facts: (1) people with fibromyalgia have a much lower level of fitness than those without, and (2) many people with fibromyalgia experience considerable improvement in their condition following a period of fitness training.

THE IMPORTANT ROLE OF ARTHRITIS FOUNDATIONS
In many countries, including Australia, there are professionally managed arthritis associations. The Arthritis Foundation of Australia, the peak body in Australia, focuses on advocacy and fundraising, and there are affiliate foundations in every state and territory. In addition to organising educational and information programs the affiliate foundations hold exercise classes in tai chi and hydrotherapy. There are also programs for chronic disease especially tailored for people with arthritis, such as the Arthritis Self-Management Course. Both the Tai Chi and Chronic Disease Management Programs are scientifically based and there is good evidence for their effectiveness. Information can be obtained from the Arthritis Australia-wide information line on 1800 011 041 or from the website at www.arthritisfoundation.com.au.

Some of the exercises in this book make use of resistance bands (see Chapter 12). If you've used these already with little or no difficulty then you may want to progress to other resistant band exercises or even to dumb-bells and/or weight machines. The resistance training and cardiovascular training programs outlined in this book should be seen as a natural progression from the Arthritis Self-Management Course and similar programs. Bear in mind that there are four functional classifications for people with arthritis:

Class 1.   Complete ability to carry on all usual duties without a high level of pain or discomfort.

Class 2.   Adequate ability for normal activities despite the handicap, discomfort or limited motion at one or more joints.

Class 3.   Ability limited to little or none of the duties of usual occupational self-care.

Class 4.   Totally incapacitated, bedridden or confined to a wheelchair, with little or no self-care.

Courses such as the Arthritis Self-Management Course have to accommodate the needs of participants in all these functional classes, while the programs outlined in this book only cater for people with arthritis in Class 1 through to Class 3. The book's programs will extend what you've done in such courses and offer you the opportunity to enhance your strength, fitness and independence.

THE BOTTOM LINE

Exercise is as beneficial for people with arthritis as it is for healthy people, and probably more so.

8 Why should I
exercise?

> *'The whole of science is nothing
> more than a refinement of
> everyday thinking.'*
>
> ALBERT EINSTEIN

Why should I exercise? At first this may seem like a silly question
with an obvious answer: 'If I don't exercise I'll gain weight and if I
gain weight I run the risk of falling prey to one of those horrors
described in Chapter 2'. True—but do you know why the need for
this has arisen?

Physical training, gyms and a focus on health are all relatively new
phenomena in society. There was a time not very long ago when
gyms were an absolute rarity, no-one bothered about physical
training and no-one thought much about what they ate. What
happened to change all of this? What happened was that people
started dying—young. It happened because the industrial revolution,
followed by the technological revolution followed by the microchip
has meant that as life has become more and more sophisticated we've
had to do less and less to accomplish the activities of daily living.
Why walk or cycle when you can drive, why get up to press a button
when you've got a remote, why wash clothes or dishes when you've
got a machine, why play sports when you can watch, why play silly
outdoor games with your kids or grandchildren when they're quite
happy 'exercising' their fingers on a video game?

Our lifestyle may have changed but physically we are no different
from our ancestors of 50000 years ago. Think of what they had to do
to survive! Their whole life was one physical workout—with a bit of
danger thrown in for good measure. It's great that technology and
computers have made our lives so much easier but the flipside is that

we're now in as much danger from underactivity as our ancestors were from the activities they had to undertake in order to survive. In 1996 the United States Surgeon General reported that only 15% of US adults participated in physical activities of sufficient intensity and regularity to meet the minimum requirements of the American College of Sports Medicine for the improvement or maintenance of fitness. Yet our muscles, bones, ligaments, tendons and cardiovascular system need the same sort of upkeep and training to ensure our survival as did our hunting ancestors tens of thousands of years ago. And because we're living longer we may need an even greater upkeep. This is why we need to exercise.

WHAT IF MY WEIGHT HASN'T CHANGED FOR 20 YEARS OR MORE?

There are a number of adults who feel greatly reassured by the fact that their weight hasn't changed over many years despite not having exercised. Is this a special group—a group who are genetically favoured and who don't need exercise? Sadly this is not the case. People who don't exercise but nevertheless maintain the same weight have simply substituted fat for lean body mass (muscle). Increasing age and a lack of exercise will always result in a loss of muscle, and bone. Your weight may not have changed (though your shape almost certainly will have) because you've gained fat at the expense of lean body mass. You're at the same risk as a person whose weight has increased as a result of increased body fat.

THE SOLUTION

The solution consists of resistance training (weight training or strength training) and cardiovascular training combined with a diet low in saturated fat. Depending on your inclination, this can be done at home or in a gym, but wherever you train you should think of it as a 'trading place' or stock exchange. A place where, in trading fat for muscle, you'll be exchanging a high-risk liability for a low-risk asset—and one with considerable fringe benefits. This could just be your most successful investment. Incidentally, a useful by-product of your new low-risk investment will be lower overheads (like fewer visits to the doctor, fewer drugs, less fast food, etc).

There is a good reason for combining resistance training with cardiovascular training. It works this way. By increasing your lean body mass through resistance training you increase your metabolic rate (see Chapter 4) and therefore the rate at which fat is burned. That newfound muscle will turn you into an efficient fat-burning unit. Remember what we discussed earlier. Muscle is metabolically active and fat is not. By increasing your lean body mass through resistance training you will increase your strength and your ability to benefit from cardiovascular (endurance) training. This is why the top track athletes combine their cardiovascular training with weight work. Remember those pre-Sydney 2000 Olympics TV grabs of Cathy Freeman doing barbell bench-presses with those impressively large weight plates? That wasn't some contrived promo—that's the way athletes train these days to improve their athletic performance. It seems to work!

THE BENEFITS
BETTER BODY SHAPE AND INCREASED STRENGTH
The benefits of resistance training are no different for men and women, and the menopause does not appear to alter the strength response to resistance training. Resistance training will reduce your body fat, increase your lean body mass and make you stronger. Remember when we said that it wasn't necessary to first check on a chart to know if somebody was fat or overweight—that it's something you just recognise because, by its very nature, fatty tissue doesn't hold its shape—it bulges and it flops around. Well, muscle, on the other hand, is firm and will enhance rather than detract from your body's shape. You won't just look trimmer and stronger, this will be your new reality. In essence you'll have performed your own cosmetic surgery—without an anaesthetic. What's more, it's cheaper, it's more enjoyable and it's natural.

Some women tend to shy away from resistance training because they were brought up in an era when 'weightlifting' was seen as a macho thing—men only stuff. Women associated resistance training with bodybuilders such as Charles Atlas (now that's a long time ago) and Arnold Schwarzenegger. That's how women may visualise the end result of a weight program. It won't happen. I can almost guarantee you that the film star, TV star or sports star whose body you may have admired ('Isn't she slim—I'd love a body like that') has done resistance training—and they're not bulging with muscle. Their slim shape is not the result of some strange quirk of nature—they worked for it. Ask Oprah Winfrey. Resistance training will result in your replacing fatty tissue with muscle. Your shape will change—for the better.

INCREASED CONFIDENCE AND SELF-ESTEEM

Being fitter, trimmer and stronger will give you added confidence and increase your self-esteem. This is not a 'skin-deep' confidence, nor is it a self-esteem based on vanity. It's something that evolves gradually through your training. It's something that you earn as you prove to yourself that you have the determination to persevere through the tough times, to get up on cold mornings when you'd rather sleep in, to come back from injuries and to stick to your program. The end result is that you'll find that you can cope with life's problems more effectively. Studies indicate that older adults who exercise have a greater sense of control over their own lives, and this has been shown to be an important factor in warding off depression.

IMPROVED POSTURE, BALANCE, MOVEMENT SPEED AND FLEXIBILITY

Whatever your age, increased muscle strength will improve your flexibility—you won't become 'muscle bound'. Increased muscle strength also means that you'll have a better posture when walking, standing, moving and exercising. This will not only make you look and feel younger, it will actually increase your endurance and movement speed, because a good posture means that your muscles will be working in a more efficient way. If you're an older person, your stronger muscles will provide you with better balance and more stability, which will reduce the risk of falling. So significant a problem is this in the elderly that in Australia some public hospitals have actually established 'falls clinics'.

INCREASED METABOLIC RATE

As I've already said, muscle, unlike fat, is metabolically active. It burns kilojoules. The more muscle the higher the metabolic rate. If you put this new-found muscle to work, you'll increase your metabolic rate even more. And because you now have more muscle you'll burn more kilojoules even on the days when you're not training! You'll also find that you can eat more (of the right foods) without gaining body fat. Financial advisors speak of the 'magic of compound interest', and what I'm describing here is the compound magic of resistance training in which efficient fat burning becomes a continuous process. We can express this as a simple equation:

increased muscle = increased metabolic rate = decreased fat = healthier and longer life

REDUCED BIOLOGICAL AGE AND LONGER LIFE

This really is the bottom line, the culmination of all of the benefits of exercising. There are now a number of studies indicating that people who exercise regularly have lower biological ages than people of the same chronological age (age in calendar years) who don't exercise. This slowing down of the ageing process is possible because we know that two-thirds of the ageing process results from lifestyle choices. What's even more encouraging is that a recent (2001) study of 1300 men of average age 52 years found that the higher the level of cardiovascular fitness, the lower the risk of premature death. Conversely, those with low fitness levels had well over twice the risk of dying from any cause, and three times the risk of dying from cardiovascular disease compared with fit people. In the United States physical inactivity has been estimated to account for 12% of all deaths.

Modify your lifestyle through resistance and cardiovascular training, good diet and being a non-smoker and you can make a difference to your biological age, which is a more accurate indication of the ageing process than the number of years you've been around. Studies have also shown that, in addition to having a lower biological age, physically active people live longer and with better health.

WEIGHT LOSS

You'll *almost* certainly lose weight. 'Hang on', I imagine you're saying. 'If I do all of this resistance and cardiovascular training surely weight loss is a *certainty*?' Well, weight reduction will occur in the great majority of people, because most people are carrying extra body fat. But if you are underweight and carrying fat your weight may *increase* because you'll gain muscle at the expense of fat, and muscle is heavier than fat. The good news is that now you will look lean and firm. You'll look lean because what has increased is your lean body mass.

REDUCTION IN HEART DISEASE, DISEASES OF BLOOD VESSELS, STROKE, HIGH BLOOD PRESSURE AND DIABETES

There is now abundant research indicating that resistance training and cardiovascular training are associated with longevity as well as a better quality of life. This happens because the sort of training I am advocating has been shown to reduce risk factors for heart and blood vessel disease, stroke, high blood pressure and diabetes. We previously discussed how, because of certain dietary fats in the body's cells, older overweight adults may develop resistance to the effects of insulin, the hormone responsible for transporting sugar and amino acids into cells. Published studies suggest that insulin resistance may also result from reduced levels of physical activity. Resistance training has been shown to increase the efficiency of the action of insulin, leading to lower blood insulin levels in middle-aged and older people and thus preventing diabetes.

One study showed that resistance training reduces blood pressure in adults. A spin-off of this is that you're less likely to require drugs, or at least less of them.

REDUCED RISK OF CANCER

Scientific studies tell us that exercise reduces the risk of breast cancer, ovarian cancer and bowel cancer. We're not absolutely certain how this works but it may relate to the fact that exercise reduces excess body fat, which is known to be a risk factor for these cancers. Resistance training has also been shown to speed up the movement of food through the bowel, and this may be another mechanism for reducing the risk of bowel cancer. It has been known for some time that the use of oral contraceptives protects women against ovarian cancer. It's only recently been found that women who engage in high levels of physical activity have a significantly reduced risk of ovarian cancer, equivalent to the reduced risk encountered in women taking oral contraceptives.

REDUCED SYMPTOMS OF ARTHRITIS

As we discussed in Chapter 7, there are a number of types of arthritis. In the commonest type, osteoarthritis (degenerative joint disease), it is usually involvement of the weight-bearing joints (hips, knees and ankles) that is associated with the greatest disability. We know that excess weight aggravates osteoarthritis and in many cases it is the main cause. Weight reduction through exercise will lessen the load on osteoarthritic joints. In those of you who do not have osteoarthritis in your weight-bearing joints, the risk of developing it will be reduced by weight loss. However, even more important than weight loss is the fact that by strengthening the leg muscles you will provide stability to your weight-bearing joints, which will further reduce the risk of developing osteoarthritis. And in those who already have osteoarthritis the improvement in joint stability will minimise the discomfort of arthritis and the disability.

In the not too distant past, doctors routinely advised patients with osteoarthritis in their weight-bearing joints to avoid exercise.

This is no longer the case. We will cover this in further detail in Part 2 of this book.

PREVENTING AND REDUCING THE RISKS OF OSTEOPOROSIS

Osteoporosis is a condition in which bones become thinner and more fragile, mainly as the result of loss of calcium. The most vulnerable are women, particularly after the menopause. Men can also be affected but it's a much slower process because men start off with bigger and thicker bones and have to lose a whole lot more calcium before they are at risk of having brittle bones.

The risk in osteoporosis is that fractures (breaks) can occur with minimal trauma. All bones are vulnerable, particularly the bones of the spine, ribs and hips. These fractures can be and usually are devastating. They are both painful and deforming. In old people a fractured hip may lead to death. The good news is that resistance training can significantly reduce the risk of osteoporosis and the risk of falling.

Once upon a time it was standard practice to advise women to walk to beat osteoporosis. We now know that walking has little benefit in the prevention of osteoporosis. We do know that to prevent osteoporosis requires resistance training or high-impact aerobics— activities that place stress on muscle and bone, which is the only way to stimulate the bone sufficiently to retain calcium and make more bone. In the over-40 age group and in people with arthritis, resistance training is preferred because it is safer than high-impact aerobics.

A six-month study on women compared the effects of high-intensity resistance training to walking. It was found that those women in the high-intensity resistance training group maintained bone density while the walking group actually lost bone density. This study also found that people with diseases of the arteries of the legs (caused by fatty plaques) experienced an improvement in muscle strength with resistance training and were able to walk greater distances and for longer periods of time.

Walking, it seems, is too gentle and does not place sufficient stress on bone to prevent osteoporosis. Long-distance running may pose a particular risk to women; it is a fact, for example, that highly trained long-distance women runners frequently stop menstruating. This is known as amenorrhoea and it significantly increases the risk of osteoporosis. Also, long-distance running tends to reduce lean body mass, and this has a negative effect on the metabolic rate.

IMPROVED PAIN CONTROL

Resistance and cardiovascular training increases the body's production of a range of hormones that are known to have beneficial effects. These hormones include human growth hormone, endorphins and encephalins (which affect mood and pain tolerance). This is one reason why physical training forms such an important part of treatment in patients with chronic pain problems.

REDUCING BRAIN AGEING, INCREASING LIFE

Physical activity does many things to the mind. Several studies have demonstrated that regular physical training can postpone age-related declines in mental processing speed and improve reaction time. We also know that people who remain intellectually active live longer. One study found that increasing blood flow to the brain through exercise improved clarity of thought and memory.

REDUCED ANXIETY AND DEPRESSION

Studies have shown that people in training programs experience a reduction in anxiety. Resistance training and cardiovascular training may work in much the same way as meditation does, by taking your focus away from stressful thoughts. When you revisit these things after a good workout you may be surprised to find you have a different perspective on issues that were previously stressing you out. If you're going through the process of trying to sort out a work or personal problem requiring a decision, it's not a bad strategy to postpone the decision until after a solid workout.

The incidence of depression is known to increase with age. It has been found that the cause may in part be a decline in physical activity. There are now several studies that have shown that regular exercise reduces depression. In one study patients previously on antidepressants were able to cease medication.

IMPROVED SLEEP
An improvement in your fitness and your strength through regular training will enhance the quality and quantity of your sleep, whatever your age. You'll sleep more deeply and wake more rested.

IMPROVED SEX LIFE
Studies indicate that in older men resistance training increases testosterone levels and improves libido. In men and women the confidence that comes with having an improved body image and from being healthier will also improve your sex life.

IMPROVED QUALITY OF LIFE
I suspect that after reading about all the potential benefits of exercise some of you who may never have previously exercised may be wondering how you managed to survive so long without exercise! Living is not just about surviving—that happens (for a while anyway), despite what we do or don't do. It's about quality of life— and if you want this it's yours for the taking.

THE RISKS
I'm not going to throw cliches at you like 'life is a risk'. When we consider 'risk' before we embark on an action we usually go through the process, either at a conscious or unconscious level, of weighing the risks against the needs or benefits of our actions. So let's have a look at the risks.

MUSCLE INJURY
A muscle 'strain' describes an injury that occurs when the muscle is working within its normal range. A muscle 'sprain' describes an

injury to muscle that is stretched beyond its normal range. Such injuries may occur when exercising muscles that are 'cold', using poor exercise technique or using weights that are too heavy. These risks will be minimised by following the proper stretching routine (Chapter 11) and by following the 'principles of resistance training' (Chapter 10).

OVERBULKING
This is not a real risk, although it may be a perceived risk. It simply won't happen—unless of course you make it a specific goal. Invariably resistance training results in an increase in lean body mass and a decrease in body fat, giving you a leaner and stronger body rather than a bulky one.

SUDDEN DEATH
The risk of sudden death during or within 30 minutes of vigorous exercise is greater than when, say, sitting in front of your TV watching Jerry Seinfeld (perhaps not ...)—but scientific studies tell us that the absolute risk is tiny, and can be diminished even further by regular exercise. One study calculated the absolute risk as being 1 death per 1.5 million episodes of physical activity. I'll take those odds any day of the week. These are good odds of staying alive and a whole lot better than winning the lottery. And try these odds: a 1987 study showed that sedentary individuals have a 100% greater risk of fatal coronary artery disease than active individuals.

Medical research confirms what you already know or at least suspect—that the small increase in absolute risk associated with exercise is greatly outweighed by the benefits. Doctors refer to this as the 'risk to benefit ratio', and every time we offer patients any kind of treatment—be it pills, injections, operations or dietary advice—we ask ourselves 'are the benefits likely to outweigh the potential risks?' I can tell you that as far as exercise goes the benefits so outweigh the risks it's a no-contest.

RISK MINIMISATION

If you have a heart condition, high blood pressure, a history of unexplained chest pain or dizziness or a high blood cholesterol level, or you are on regular medication for whatever reason, it's advisable to have a check-up before starting a training program. If none of the above applies to you but you've had a sedentary lifestyle, or are significantly overweight or have never trained before, then a check-up is also advisable. If you have any concerns at all, go for a check-up anyway. This will put your mind at ease and will stop you from holding back because of nagging doubts about your health status. It's all about risk minimisation. In Chapter 10 we'll discuss in detail a range of specific techniques that will not only minimise the risk of injury while doing resistance training but will ensure that you get the most out of your training time. In Chapter 15 we will discuss how to minimise the risk and maximise the benefits while undertaking cardiovascular training, by monitoring your heart rate.

To ensure a gradual approach to training, my program starts at Level 1 (low intensity), progressing through to Level 2 (moderate intensity) and finally to Level 3 (high intensity). For older adults and for people with severe arthritis there is a preparatory starting level which I've called Pre-Level 1 (low intensity). Later I'll explain in detail how to judge at which level you should begin both your resistance training program and your cardiovascular program, and if or when you should put yourself up to the next level.

MAKING THE COMMITMENT

We make a commitment to go to work and trade our labour and expertise for cash so we can buy the essentials of life and, with what's left, the luxuries. What I'm suggesting is just as important because if you don't have your health you won't be able to trade your labour and expertise, or at least for not as long as you would have hoped. And what if you're already retired? Someone once said 'You're a long time dead'. Now we're saying 'You're a long time retired'. We are part of the longer life revolution. We need to prepare ourselves.

The first and major commitment is to factor your training time into your life's schedule just as you factor in going to work. You should view your training session as important as a doctor's appointment. If you have retired you are still going to have to make time from all the things you're already doing. This could be gardening, golfing, bowling, fishing, volunteer or charity work, part-time work, hobbies, reading or looking after your spouse. Everyone is busy. Perhaps that's why you're reading this book. You're looking to find some way to fit it all in.

By definition busy people have commitments. It's a good habit to have. It may give you the edge in making the one commitment that will enhance your busy life. One piece of advice: you should not find your training commitment grossly inconvenient because in the end it may be the inconvenience that defeats you. It is far better to first adjust things in your life to enable you to commit rather than hoping 'things will work out'. If you are working perhaps you could get up slightly earlier to start your exercise program and then start work a half hour later, or perhaps start work earlier than usual and leave earlier to fit in an afternoon training session. The good news is that it gets easier as you progress through the program. But remember the promise you made to yourself—eight weeks—hang in there. By then you will be fitter and stronger and your energy levels will have increased. You will find you can do a whole lot more and fit it all into your day.

THE BOTTOM LINE

There is as yet no known alternative way of maintaining good health other than by exercising.

Chapter 9

To gym or
not to gym?

> *'Senility is when one goes about doing only that towards which one is most inclined.'*

YAMAMOTO TSUNETOMO,
THE BOOK OF THE SAMURAI (HAGAKURE)

ARE GYMS OK FOR OLDER ADULTS?

People who have never been to a gym are sometimes frightened by the thought of going to one. It's not that gyms are frightening places, it's just that we all have a healthy fear of the unknown. As we get older we may become less sure of ourselves physically and this adds to our concerns. Perhaps you mistakenly think that younger people resent the presence of older adults in a gym? Perhaps you think that going to a gym is not 'acting your age' or that others may think this? This sort of stereotyping may have existed 20 or 30 years ago but not now.

What you may not know is that fitness trainers really enjoy working with or advising older adults. Why is this? It's because they understand the sorts of challenges that you've had to overcome in attending the gym. Just being there tells the fitness trainer that you are motivated. He or she also knows that you will make faster progress than a younger person and that this will be apparent within a matter of eight to 12 weeks. If you decide to attend a gym and to follow the programs outlined in this book, you will find trainers all too willing to lend a hand and give advice.

There are now numerous gyms in most cities and towns that cater specifically for older adults. This is all part of a modern-day revolution energised by the growing awareness of the health benefits of exercise for people of all ages. People with a severe disability may benefit from personal instruction rather than being in a class situation. For addresses of gyms check out the 'Further Resources' at the end of this book.

Some older adults are more comfortable attending classes with people of a similar age group—this also provides the opportunity to make social contacts, and in fact many gyms hold social functions for their members. Other older adults prefer to train with younger members.

Training is important but it's not serious. It's fun and it's healthy.

THE EQUIPMENT

Another thing that puts some people off gyms is being surrounded by all that equipment, and having the feeling that you just don't know how to use it all and will look foolish. Forget about it. This book will show you the correct exercise techniques and how to use the weight machines. As far as the cardiovascular machines are concerned, almost every first-timer (of any age) has asked a gym instructor how to operate these machines and set the programs. That's what the instructors are there for. They welcome enquiries. If you didn't ask them, they'd have nothing to do. Usually when you first go to a gym the instructor will show you how to operate everything anyway.

SELF-IMAGE

I've found that one of the main reasons for people not wanting to go to a gym is their self-image. Overweight people are sometimes embarrassed going to a gym and putting on gym gear. Yet they shouldn't be. There is a distinct advantage in being overweight when you start your resistance training program: your gains will be greater and more dramatic.

ARE GYMS OK FOR PEOPLE WITH ARTHRITIS?

People with arthritis may feel embarrassed about going to a gym because they feel that gyms are only for 'healthy' people. Well, I have news for you. I have been into gyms all over the world and I'm still waiting to see the notice above the door that reads 'Healthy people only—enter here'. Gyms are for everybody, whatever your age, size, arthritic status or disability status. They are a place where everyone can go to help themselves. By taking yourself to the gym you are taking the first, important step. You won't be strange or out of place. I can tell you the great majority of gym users admire and welcome anyone prepared to make the effort to improve themselves. Mostly people who use gyms are on a time schedule—like you. They are so focused on what they're doing they pay very little attention to anyone else. And the people you may see looking so at ease in a gym environment weren't born there! They had to make a start just like everybody else.

THE CONVENIENCE FACTOR

I like gyms because they make getting healthy a little easier. They have everything you need, including machines for cardiovascular work, a range of free weights, pin-loaded or hydraulic weight machines, resistance bands and, of course, instructors who'll provide helpful advice. Also, buying a membership is a motivation for using what you've bought. Another motivator is being among people looking to do exactly what you're about to do—exploring self-potential and getting healthier while doing it. You may find that working out at home will be limited by your not having all the equipment. I also think it's that bit harder to motivate yourself to work out in isolation. Perhaps there isn't a gym close to your home or workplace so that getting to a gym may be really inconvenient or even impossible. It's not the end of the world! For a small outlay you can purchase the basics (see 'Further Resources').

PREVENTING GYM FALLOUT ('DROPOUT DISEASE')

One of the prime reasons for 'gym fallout' is boredom. The programs I have devised provide variety and flexibility and the opportunity to progress from level to level. I hope boredom will never be a problem.

Another reason for gym fallout is the absence of a goal and a structured plan to turn this goal into a reality. Many people who decide to go to a gym do so because it seems like a 'good idea' or because it's the 'thing to do' or because they know someone who goes. That may be good enough to get you there but it's not enough to keep you there. My programs provide a plan, goal opportunities and a strategy to help you achieve your goals, irrespective of whether these are your own personal goals or the suggested training levels detailed in Chapters 13 and 16. In Chapter 18 we'll discuss the all-important issue of how to set goals and how to go about turning those goals into reality.

Some of you may prefer to make a start at home so that you are familiar with the exercises before venturing into a gym—that's OK too. But please don't avoid going to a gym because you feel your body is not fit for public viewing! Don't try to 'trim down' before hitting the gym. You're making things hard on yourself. I can tell you that if the only people going to gyms were those who were trim, taut and terrific, gyms wouldn't exist—they'd all go bust (no pun intended). And remember you have a huge advantage over 90% of people going to the gym for the first time. You have a plan to achieve your goal and a strategy to fulfil it.

THE BOTTOM LINE

Gyms are not a habitat solely for the young and fit. They are for everybody, whatever your age, size, shape, arthritic status or disability status.

Chapter **10** Principles of resistance training

> *'Be true to the thought of the moment and avoid distraction. Other than continuing to exert yourself, enter into nothing else, but go to the extent of living single thought by single thought.'*
>
> YAMAMOTO TSUNETOMO,
> *THE BOOK OF THE SAMURAI* (HAGAKURE)

Think of this chapter as the 'ABC' of resistance (strength) training. It should be read carefully. The principles described will provide the foundation of what I hope for you will be a lifelong journey in safe and enjoyable strength training. I won't be describing anything that's difficult to understand. The appeal of resistance training is its simplicity, which is probably why so few people are involved. People generally seem to be attracted by complexity and exclusivity, which is not what this is all about. Focus always on the journey—the destination will follow.

Resistance training can involve lifting free weights (dumb-bells, barbells, EZ or 'curly' bar), using weight machines (pin loaded or hydraulic) or resistance bands, and lifting or moving your own body weight (push-ups, chin-ups, sit-ups and dips).

WEIGHT TALK
Barbell: A long bar on the ends of which weight plates are held in place with 'collars'.
Dumb-bell: A short bar weighted at each end with a roundish knob; dumb-bells are usually used in pairs.

Reps (repetitions): This is the number of times you perform the exercise (lifting and lowering the weight is one repetition). In some exercises, dumb-bells or other weights are lifted simultaneously. In others they are lifted using first one arm and then the other, or one leg and then the other. If the exercise requires '10 reps' and you are alternating arms (or legs) then you need to do 10 reps with *each* arm (or leg).

Set: A sequence of consecutive reps performed without a rest is known as a 'set'. For example, you may do 10 reps per set and do two or three sets (or more) of an exercise for a particular muscle group.

Weight machine: This describes an apparatus that operates on a hydraulic or pulley mechanism. For 'pin-loaded' machines the resistance (the weight being lifted) is determined by placing a steel pin into whatever weight you decide to lift.

PS—BEFORE YOU BEGIN

Normally, 'PS' appears at the end of a letter and stands for 'postscript'. In resistance training it stands for 'position and stability' (and since this must be right *before* you do resistance training, you could say it also stands for 'pre-script').

Position and stability involve three elements:

(1) your position in relation to the position of the weight, weight machine, resistance band, fitness ball, etc

(2) the position of these pieces of equipment in relation to you, and

(3) most importantly, the position and stability of your body. When (in Chapter 12) I ask you to 'set yourself' for an exercise I'm reminding you to pay attention to position and stability.

HOW DO WE POSITION AND STABILISE THE BODY?

There are five steps to getting 'PS' right. Think 'head to pelvis' for all starting positions:

(1) Flex your upper neck by tucking in your chin, and relax your jaw.

(2)   Relax your shoulders.

(3)   'Stand tall' by elevating your sternum (breast bone).

(4)   Brace and stabilise your lower back by simultaneously drawing your belly button up and backwards towards your spine and tilting your pubic bone towards your chin—to do this make a 'pelvic thrust' and maintain this position. (As you'll see in Chapters 12 and 17 this can take practice!)

(5)   If the resistance training exercise is to be performed standing, slightly bend the knees while still 'standing tall'.

This may appear a little complicated but believe me it's not. After two or three sessions it will become automatic and you won't have to consciously think about these five steps. And by getting the 'PS' right you'll maximise the benefits of the exercise and ensure that the exercise will be done safely.

WHAT'S THE CORRECT EXERCISE SEQUENCE?

As a general rule you should work larger muscle groups before smaller muscle groups, e.g. lats/back before chest, chest before shoulders, shoulders before triceps, triceps before biceps, quadriceps before hamstrings, hamstrings before calves (see Chapter 12 for a diagram of all these muscles). The reason for this is very simple. Smaller muscle groups help stabilise the larger ones during resistance training. They also tire more easily. If you've exhausted the smaller muscles by exercising them before the larger muscles you'll find that the large muscles will fatigue more quickly and you may struggle to finish your routine.

THE RIGHT WAY TO LIFT WEIGHTS
BREATHING

Always breathe *out* on the lifting phase ('power phase') of the exercise and breathe *in* on the lowering phase ('relaxation phase'). Beginners often breathe in or even hold their breath while lifting, which can increase the blood pressure unnecessarily and this could be dangerous. It will also reduce your power. Imagine as you're breathing out while pushing the weight away from your body, that you're blowing the weight away from your body. This 'breathing out'principle on the lifting phase is employed by martial artists when punching or kicking and is sometimes accompanied by a shout or 'kiyai'. This is not just designed to intimidate the opponent, it provides the focus for an explosion of power. Sometimes in resistance training when you're struggling to complete a set you may need to draw on this principle to complete your lift (don't shout too loudly, though—you'll frighten your fellow exercisers).

FORM (OR TECHNIQUE)

I cannot overemphasise the importance of good 'form', or technique, in resistance training. This is a pet theme of mine. This is not because it's important to look good or even to look like you know what you're doing. It's because poor form will slow your progress and can result in injury. It may turn out to be the one thing that prevents you from reaching your goal or at least from reaching your goal as quickly as you would like.

Let's take a step back. In the lifting (power) phase of resistance training the muscles are shortening to achieve the lift (even when the weight is being pushed further *away* from your body, as in a dumb-bell chest press or dumb-bell shoulder press, the muscles doing the work are shortening). In the lowering (relaxation) phase the muscles are lengthening. Almost everyone focuses on the lifting phase and consequently almost everyone tries to lift the heaviest weight they possibly can, believing that this is the best way to build muscles and strength quickly. This is incorrect. Scientific studies tell us that it is the lowering phase that is more important in the building of strength. Exactly! The very opposite of what seems so obvious.

Why or how does this happen? Remember we discussed earlier that for muscle remodelling and building to take place it is first necessary that the muscle fibres undergo a process of 'microdamage'. This process appears to be greatest in the course of the lowering phase of muscle contraction, hence its pivotal role in muscle and strength building.

What can we learn from this scientific observation? We can learn that by lifting and lowering a weight in good form we can make more progress than by lifting a heavier weight with poor form, e.g. driving it up too quickly and then lowering it too quickly without control. An important additional bonus of good form is that there is much less risk of injury. This is because good form means you're in control of the weight.

If you find it is difficult to complete your sets in a controlled fashion with the weights you are currently lifting and lowering, then the weights may be too heavy for you. Just reduce your weights by 5 pounds (roughly 2.5 kilograms, though you'll find that many gyms, have still not gone metric!). You will reduce the risk of injury and will make more rapid progress. Heavy weights that are not being properly controlled increase the risk of injury because of stresses on the ligaments and tendons, *and* because the weight is too heavy you'll end up doing 'cheat sets'. This means using other muscle groups and joints to complete the lift, such as throwing your weight backwards while straining to do a barbell biceps curl (see Chapter 12 for a description of this and other exercises) when the weight is too heavy for you. You may 'complete' the process of getting the weight up, but because you've 'cheated' you won't gain full benefit from the exercise. This will slow your progress and increase the risk of injury. This is such an important point that if in the course of an exercise you can't complete a rep or a set without compromising form and/or body position and stability, then you should immediately abort the exercise. You can then reduce the weight before completing your set.

RANGE OF EXERCISE MOVEMENT

Wherever possible the muscle group being exercised should be taken through its full range in order to get the maximum benefit from the exercise. When doing a dumb-bell biceps curl, for example, fully extend the elbow at the end of the lowering phase and then fully flex the elbow at the end of the lifting phase. The three exceptions to this rule are:

(1)   where the exercise specifically requires that the joint not be fully extended for safety reasons, e.g. in machine leg presses it's important not to fully extend the knees when pressing the weight because this results in too much weight being borne directly through the knee joint, which could injure the joint

(2)   in people with arthritis who have a limited range of joint movement as a result of joint damage or inflammation, and

(3)   in 'hypermobile' people, i.e. those with excessively mobile joints and ligaments, who should work only in the mid-range.

RHYTHM WITHOUT THE BLUES

All movement has a rhythm or cadence to it. Lifting and lowering weights is no different. I've experimented with a range of rhythms and have found the most effective lift to lowering ratio is 2:3. Count 1-2 on the lifting phase then pause for 1 second at the completion of the lift before counting 1-2-3 when lowering the weight, pause for 1 second then repeat the process for your next rep. This is a rhythm that won't give you the blues through injury. It will give you control, whether you're using dumb-bells, a barbell, a weight machine or resistance bands.

WHEN TO EXERCISE

While exercising at almost any time is good, there are now scientific studies that suggest that exercising in the fasting state (this usually means in the morning) enhances the fat-burning process.

It is not advisable to exercise soon after eating a large meal. Leaving aside the feeling of discomfort from a stomach full of food, older adults may experience reflux symptoms. There are also studies that suggest there is an increased risk of heart attack in older adults who exercise after consuming a large meal.

It is also unwise to exercise if you have a heavy dose of the flu, because you won't be able to exercise to your full potential and, more importantly, you may place an undue strain on your heart—no matter what your age. (It's also not considerate to your fellow gym members.)

HOW OFTEN TO DO RESISTANCE TRAINING

It's much easier to do resistance training three times a week than twice a week and very much easier to train twice a week than once a week. This is because the more often you train the faster you'll progress. As you increase in strength your exercising becomes easier and more enjoyable.

Ultimately, how often you do resistance training is really up to you, but the more you do the greater your progress will be—up to a point. This is because muscles grow in size and strength through a process of microdamage and require 48 hours for the repair and growth process to take place. For this reason, resistance training for the *same muscle group* should therefore not be undertaken more than three times a week. This does not mean that you have to take to your bed in between resistance training sessions. But it does mean, for example, that on the day after a full upper body resistance training workout you can do a lower body resistance training workout or a cardiovascular session but not another upper body workout.

HOW LONG PER SESSION?

The short answer is: until you've finished what you set out to do. In Chapter 14 you will see that Level 1 resistance training sessions take roughly 30 minutes, Level 2 sessions around 40 minutes and Level 3 sessions 50 minutes or longer. Older adults (over 60 years) and people with arthritis may initially be able to tolerate only low intensity, short-duration sessions lasting no more than 10 minutes.

HOW DO I KNOW WHEN TO INCREASE MY LIFTING WEIGHTS?

When you find that you can complete your sets of a particular exercise with no feeling of stress to the muscles, then the weight is too light for you. Your strength has increased—the weight hasn't changed! Now increase your reps by two per set. When you find you can do 12 reps with ease, increase your weights by between 2.5 pounds and 5 pounds and reduce the reps by two.

SAFETY FIRST—WHEN TO USE A 'SPOTTER'

If you're undertaking high-intensity (Level 3) resistance training you'll need to lift heavy weights. In this case a training partner or gym instructor is necessary to act as a 'spotter' or facilitator. This is advisable where there is a danger of losing control of the weight, or when you may need help (facilitation) to complete your set, e.g. barbell chest press, dumb-bell chest flys, cable lats pull-down, EZ bar triceps extension.

WHAT TO EXPECT

You can expect to feel some muscle soreness. If you haven't previously done resistance training, start gradually to minimise this effect. Note that it may be most noticeable the next day or even the day after that. This is quite normal. Don't be alarmed, the soreness will disappear with further training. Muscle soreness is not a reason to miss a session but you should spend a little longer on your stretch-up. By eight weeks you can expect to feel worthwhile benefits, such as increased strength and (depending on exercise intensity) improved body shape. If you were overweight to start, you will probably lose some weight, and if you were underweight you are likely to gain some weight through muscle development (see Chapter 8).

People with arthritis will need to distinguish between muscle soreness and joint pain. Usually it's not too difficult to distinguish between pain that is located in a joint from pain in the surrounding muscle. If it is *joint* pain, then you need to modify your training, or see your doctor.

WHAT NOT TO EXPECT

Do not immediately expect to find exercise a wonderful, fulfilling experience! It can take up to eight weeks before you develop strength and fitness sufficiently to be able to focus on the pleasurable aspects of your training.

You'll find that the first eight weeks are going to be your testing time. You will need to focus on your goals and on the knowledge that your new training (and eating) program will develop health benefits that will continue into the long term, even if they're not immediately apparent to you. Think of it this way: you've made your investment and are still waiting for your first dividend—which is guaranteed. Don't sell the stock before you receive your first dividend.

To further sustain yourself during the testing first eight weeks, you can reward yourself after workouts by booking a massage or having a soak in a spa. And if you're finding things a struggle this is the time when it's often helpful to discuss your concerns with an exercise partner or fitness trainer.

Hopefully your partner, family and friends will be supportive of your new training regime but some may not be, for whatever reason. You should mentally prepare yourself for negative comments and try to avoid discussing your training with people who may be discouraging or who are unsupportive.

WHAT TO WEAR

Your training shoes are the most important and usually the most expensive piece of gear. Most people own a pair of 'joggers'. If you're going to buy new training shoes ask for 'cross-trainers', shoes which are suitable for gym work and for walking. Comfort is the key. Clothing should be light and loose fitting (see 'Further Resources'). There are now available synthetic materials that promote cooling, though they can be expensive.

WHAT ABOUT MY OTHER SPORTING INTERESTS?

Resistance training is not only compatible with other sports, these days it forms an integral part of cross-training for track and field athletes, footballers, hockey players, cricketers, boxers, martial artists, wrestlers, gymnasts, cyclists, swimmers, lacrosse players, downhill and cross-country skiers, tennis players, squash players, golfers, rowers, scullers, skydivers, archers, pistol shooters, lawn bowlers and ten-pin bowlers—everybody! This is because the increased strength, muscle control and flexibility that come with resistance training enhance the skills required in these sporting activities.

PLANNING AND EXECUTING THE TRAINING SESSION
WHAT TO THINK ABOUT BEFORE YOUR RESISTANCE TRAINING SESSION

Before going to a training session it is important to know exactly what you will be doing during your session. For example, you may be planning an upper body workout. You'll have already worked out in advance your maximum single lift per body part (see Chapter 13) and you know you'll be training with a weight that's 60–80% of your maximum single lift (this will vary depending on your training level). The weights you'll be using for each body part will soon become second nature but initially you may have to write them down on your workout sheet until they are committed to memory. If you are using one of the resistance training levels in Chapter 13, it is advisable to write down your weekly schedule so you can consult it when necessary.

WHAT TO THINK ABOUT AND FEEL DURING YOUR RESISTANCE TRAINING SESSION

There is only one 'rule': think only about what you are doing! Believe it or not, studies indicate that if you mentally focus on the muscle group(s) you are exercising and concentrate on feeling the muscle contracting, your muscle development will be enhanced. Keep 'in touch' with your body. This may be hard at first because in some cases you'll be exercising muscles you never knew you had. Persevere with it and you'll find that it gets easier. If you intend to build muscle and strength then, at various stages in your resistance training sessions, you will need to do high-intensity work. This is the only way to cause the microdamage to muscle fibres necessary for muscle and strength building. This is sometimes referred to as the 'progressive muscle overload principle'.

At some point (sooner or later) you'll find that everything is getting easier. Remember the overload principle and increase your weight and/or move on to a higher level.

A selection of gym products can be purchased from www.live-stronger-live-longer.com.

THE BOTTOM LINE

By concentrating on the important principles of position and stability, breathing technique, good form and correct rhythm, and by focusing on the muscles that are being exercised, you will achieve all of the great benefits of resistance training with minimum risk.

part 2 Getting down to it

Chapter 11   Stretching up and stretching down

> 'The average, healthy, well-adjusted adult gets up at seven-thirty in the morning feeling just plain terrible.'
>
> JEAN KERR

It has been my observation that stretching is either overlooked or given little attention, most frequently by the keenest and by the fittest exercisers. They get into the gym and can't wait to get down to it. They simply can't be bothered to stretch, or incorrectly believe that stretching is only for beginners. They do so at their peril. They may get away with it most of the time, but it only needs one catastrophe, such as a torn hamstring, to be one of the less memorable events in your training experience.

To help prevent muscle damage it is important to stretch before starting your training workout, whether it's a resistance training or cardiovascular training session. I call this the 'stretch-up', and it's really in two parts: a warm-up (on a treadmill, bike etc.) for 2 minutes and then stretches for about 6 minutes. I recommend so-called 'static' stretches, as described in this chapter, which are convenient and easy to do, and do not require a partner. Stretching has multiple benefits. It improves the range of movement and function of joints, increases tendon flexibility and reduces the risk of injury. Most importantly, recent studies indicate that stretching exercises *enhance muscle performance*. It is important when entering the gym to resist the temptation to get straight into the routine without warming and stretching up.

After your workout you should do a 'stretch-down', and it too has two parts: a 'cool-down' for 2 minutes, then the same stretches as before for about 6 minutes. The purpose of the stretch-down is to give your cardiovascular system the opportunity to accommodate gradually to a lowering of its workload. This will prevent abrupt falls in blood pressure.

If you're a Pre-Level 1 exerciser, or Level 1 exerciser over 60 years of age, then for your first six weeks of training it is advisable to spend as long as 12–15 minutes on stretching before starting your cardiovascular or resistance training.

WARMING UP AND STRETCHING SAFELY

Our ideas of stretching have changed in recent years. Once we were advised to do our stretches 'cold'—immediately before we started our exercise routine—in the belief that this would reduce the risk of muscle, ligament and tendon strains and sprains. Now we know that by stretching 'cold' muscles before exercise we can actually do them more damage than by doing no stretches at all! (This was once described to me as trying to bend dry spaghetti.) There's a very simple way to avoid this:

(1)   Before you do your 'stretching', do a gentle pre-stretch cardiovascular warm-up—2 minutes on the treadmill, cross-trainer, exercise bike, stepper or rower—and only then do your stretches.

(2)   Control your stretching. The key to avoiding injury while stretching is to gradually increase the stretch so that your muscles, ligaments and tendons can accommodate it. Once you reach the point in your stretch when you feel the 'pull' in your muscles, pause at that point for 5 seconds before increasing the stretch a little more and holding it for the remainder of your stretch time, usually 20 to 30 seconds. Avoid the common habit of 'bouncing' at the end of the stretch, i.e. bobbing back and forth to get that extra stretch. This may cause injury. We'll keep returning to this important point of control while stretching and while exercising.

STRETCHES PERFORMED WHILE SITTING

Start your stretch routine seated on a floor mat. (Remember to be warmed up before you start these stretches.)

1. Inner thigh
(adductor muscle) **stretch.**
Sit upright with your feet opposing each other, grasp your ankles and use your elbows to ease your knees towards the floor. Feel the 'pull' in your inner thighs and hold the position for 20 seconds. Gently relax and repeat once more.

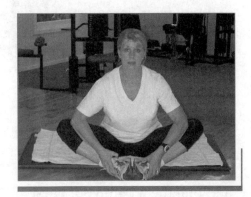

2. Hamstring stretch
Stretch out your left leg and place your right foot against your left knee (the toe of your right foot should be level with the bottom of your left knee). Reach forward with both hands and grasp the toe of your left shoe, leaning forwards at the waist while keeping your back straight, until you feel the pull in your hamstrings. Hold the position for 30 seconds. Repeat on the other leg. Remember to keep your back straight and not bend your head forward. If you can't reach your toe, lean forward as far as you can until you feel the stretch.

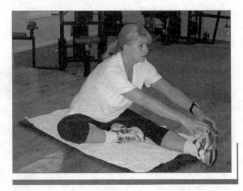

3. Hip and low back stretch

While lying flat on your back ('supine'), lock both hands behind your right leg just behind the knee and pull your flexed leg to your chest. Try to keep your back flat on the floor and keep your left leg extended straight out. Hold the position for 20 seconds. Repeat with the other leg. Now, while still lying on your back, lock both hands behind your knees and pull them onto your chest. Hold for 20 seconds.

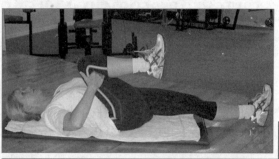

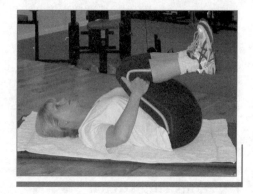

4. Lower back (lumbar) mobilisation

While lying on your back, bend your right knee and with your left hand grasp it, then pull it across to the left-hand side of your body. At the same time, try to keep your right shoulder flat on the ground with your right arm at 90° to your body. Your head should be rotated to the right side and you should be looking at your right hand. Hold for 20 seconds, then repeat for the other leg. This is a particularly good exercise for stretching the supporting (facet) joints in the lower back.

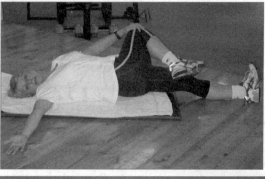

STRETCHES PERFORMED WHILE STANDING

Finish your stretch routine with some standing stretches.

5. Quadriceps stretch

The quadriceps are the muscles at the front of your thigh. To stretch them, lift your left foot and grasp the toe of your left foot with your right hand, then pull your left foot towards your right buttock. Keep the left knee alongside the right. Feel the pull in the front of your quadriceps and hold for 20 seconds. Repeat this for the other leg. Keep your back straight and avoid leaning forwards during this stretch .

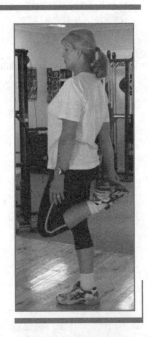

6. Shoulder stretch No 1

With your right hand, grasp your left upper arm under the triceps (muscles at the back of the upper arm) and pull your left arm across your chest while keeping your left elbow slightly bent. Hold this position for 20 seconds. Repeat for the other arm. This exercise will mobilise your acromioclavicular joint. As we get older we really do feel the 'tightness' in our shoulders. This is because our acromioclavicular joints become stiffer and our rotator cuffs become worn. For the over-40-year-olds, shoulder injuries are very, very common. Treat your shoulders with respect.

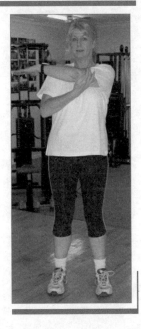

7. Shoulder Stretch No 2

Stand upright with your feet shoulder width apart. Intertwine your fingers, with the elbows straight, and gently try to raise your arms towards your head. Try to hold your stretch for 20 seconds. This is an excellent stretching exercise for both the shoulders and upper arms.

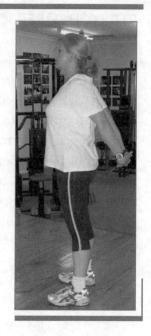

Chapter **12**   How to
do the
resistance exercises

'To practise whatever you do the
same way all the time is a must.
To practise a technique only half-
heartedly builds bad habits and
lessens one's practice time for the
proper technique ... remember
also that dishonesty
to oneself is bad discipline.'

MIYAMOTO MUSASHI,
THE BOOK OF FIVE RINGS

In this chapter I will describe resistance exercises that are suitable for over-40-year-olds and ones that are suitable for people with arthritis. In Chapter 13 I will look at the four resistance training levels in detail, then in Chapter 14 describe how the various exercises can be incorporated into a resistance training program that is suitable for your current level of strength (but be prepared to move to higher levels as you get stronger). Until you familiarise yourself with the different exercises, you may need to continually refer back to this chapter.

For free weights (barbells, dumb-bells, etc.) and/or weight machines there will usually be four exercises for each upper body muscle group and two exercises for each lower body muscle group. This is because your legs will get exercised during the cardiovascular workouts (treadmill, exercise bike, rower, stepper, versa climber, cross-trainer etc.), which are dealt with in Chapters 15 and 16.

THE MUSCLES OF THE BODY

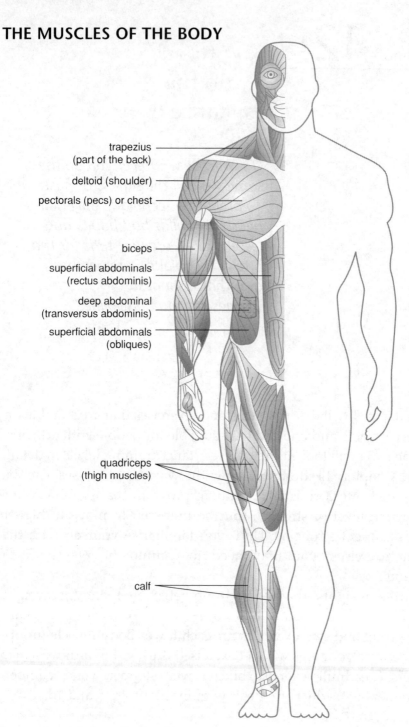

trapezius
(part of the back)

deltoid (shoulder)

pectorals (pecs) or chest

biceps

superficial abdominals
(rectus abdominis)

deep abdominal
(transversus abdominis)

superficial abdominals
(obliques)

quadriceps
(thigh muscles)

calf

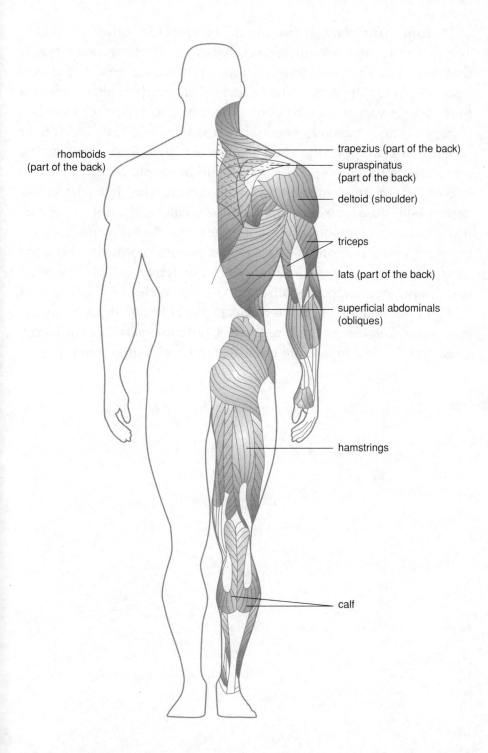

rhomboids
(part of the back)

trapezius (part of the back)

supraspinatus
(part of the back)

deltoid (shoulder)

triceps

lats (part of the back)

superficial abdominals
(obliques)

hamstrings

calf

In time you may learn about or develop other exercises. The reason for having different exercises for the same body part is that they place different stresses on the same muscle groups and may stimulate different parts of the same muscle group. It also helps you to introduce variations into your program. The variety of exercises using resistance bands is necessarily less than with free weights or weight machines, but the exercises are equally effective for muscle and strength building in older adults and in people with arthritis.

Note the method of naming the exercises. The first part of the description is the type of equipment, the second is the muscle or part being used (see previous pages for a diagram of all the muscles) and the third is the motion. Where there is possible confusion between exercises, the position (standing, seated or lying) is also described (e.g. 'dumb-bell seated shoulder press'). The codes PL1, L1, L2 and L3 that appear in brackets after an exercise indicate which levels the exercise is suitable for, i.e. Pre-Level 1 (low intensity), Level 1 (low intensity), Level 2 (moderate intensity) or Level 3 (high intensity).

FREE WEIGHTS, WEIGHT MACHINE, BODY WEIGHT AND FITNESS BALL EXERCISES

LATS/BACK

1. Cable lats pull-down (L1, L2, L3)

Start: Sit facing the lats pull-down machine with your knees under the support pads (these will stop your legs from coming up during the exercise). Hold the top of the bar with your arms wide apart and with your knuckles facing towards you. Set yourself.

The exercise: To a count of 1-2 and while breathing out pull the bar down just below your chin, pause for 1 second, then in a controlled fashion to a count of 1-2-3 and while breathing in allow the bar to return to the starting position, pause for 1 second. Repeat.

Don't pull the bar down too far.
Don't lean back.

NOTE that there is no advantage in pulling the bar down behind your head. This can be difficult for over-40-year-olds because of stiffness in the acromioclavicular joints of the neck. It can also lead to neck strain (as you crane your head forward to avoid hitting it with the bar) if you don't do it right.

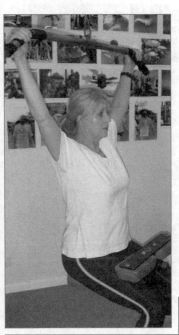

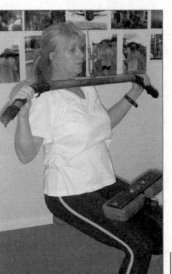

2. Cable reverse grip lats pull-down (PL1, L1, L2, L3)

Start: Sit facing the lats pull-down machine with your knees under the support pads. Grip the bar at shoulder width with your knuckles facing away from you. Set yourself.

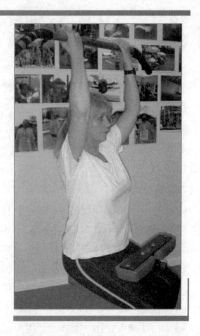

The exercise: To a count of 1-2 and while breathing out pull the bar down to your upper chest, pause for 1 second, then to a count of 1-2-3 and while breathing in allow the bar to return to its resting position, pause for 1 second. Repeat.

Don't let your elbows splay sideways.

Don't lean back.

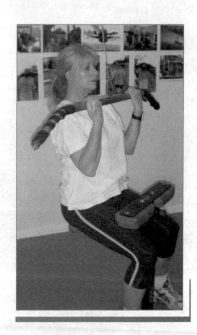

3. Dumb-bell one arm lats row (PL1, L1, L2, L3)

Start: Rest your left knee on the bench with your left arm extended and your elbow straight. You should be leaning forward with your left arm supporting your upper body weight. Your right foot should be flat on the ground. While it's not necessary to look up with this exercise, you must keep your back braced. Pick the dumb-bell off the floor with your right hand.
Set yourself.

The exercise: To a count of 1-2 and while breathing out lift the weight until your elbow will go no further, pause for 1 second, then to a count of 1-2-3 and while breathing in lower the dumb-bell to your starting position, pause for 1 second. Repeat. Complete your reps on this side before exercising the other side.

Don't rotate your back to the left to increase leverage as you pull the weight up.

Don't lift your right foot off the floor.

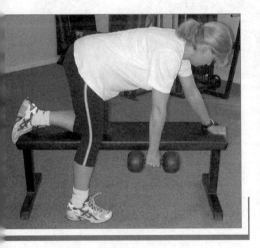
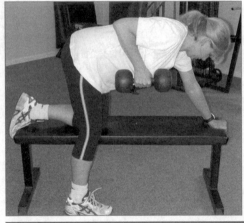

4. Dumb-bell back pull-over (L2, L3)

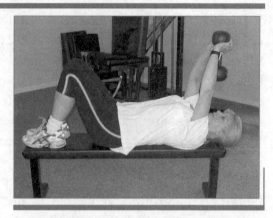

Start: Lie flat on the bench with your head close to the end of the bench and with your feet on the bench (this helps to flatten the lower back and avoid back strain). Lift the weight overhead with your arms straight and your thumbs overlapping on the dumb-bell. Set yourself.

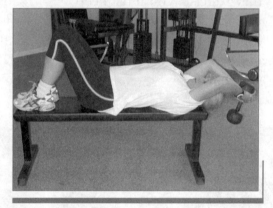

The exercise: To a count of 1-2-3 and while breathing in gently lower the weight as far as it will go, pause for 1 second, then to a count of 1-2 and while breathing out, raise the dumb-bell to your starting position, pause for 1 second. Repeat.

   Don't lift your back or bottom off the bench when lowering or raising the dumb-bell.

CHEST

1. Dumb-bell chest press (PL1, L1, L2, L3)

Start: Lie flat on the bench with your feet on the bench (remember this helps flatten out the lower back and reduces back strain). Hold the dumb-bells at chest level with the inner part of the dumb-bell in line with your shoulders and with your knuckles facing you.
Set yourself.

The exercise: To a count of 1-2 and while breathing out push the dumb-bells up in line with your chest (not in line with your shoulders) and let the dumb-bells touch at the top of the lift (this creates a 'squeeze' in the inner pecs which is good for building), pause for 1 second, then to a count of 1-2-3 and while breathing in lower the dumb-bells to your starting position, pause for 1 second. Repeat.

Don't grip the dumb-bells so tightly that your knuckles turn white—this will fatigue your forearm muscles.

NOTE that it is not necessary to fully straighten ('lock') the elbows; this exercise works the middle and lower part of the pecs.

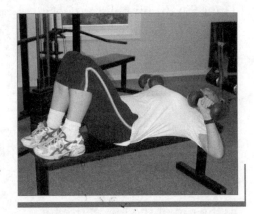

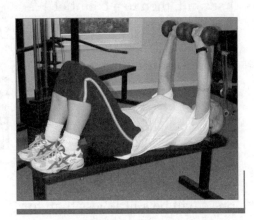

2. Dumb-bell incline chest press (PL1, L1, L2, L3)

Start: The bench should be inclined to 45° (because we're working the upper pecs—(if the incline is too low you're basically getting too close to a normal dumb-bell chest press and if it's too high you'll end up doing a shoulder press). Hold the dumb-bells at chest level with the inner part of the dumb-bells in line with your shoulders and knuckles facing you. Set yourself.

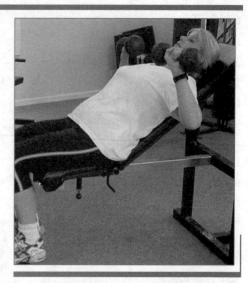

The exercise: To a count of 1-2 and while breathing out push the dumb-bells up over your upper chest and let them touch at the top of the lift, pause for 1 second, then to a count of 1-2-3 and while breathing in lower the dumb-bells to your starting position, pause for 1 second. Repeat.

Don't lift your back off the incline bench while lifting.

NOTE that it's not necessary to 'lock' the elbows; usually the weight you use for an incline press will be a little less than for a dumb-bell chest press.

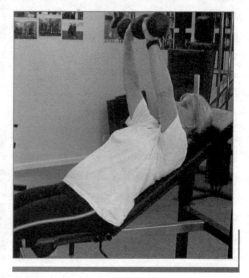

3. Dumb-bell chest flys
(PL1, L1, L2, L3)

Start: Lie flat on the bench with your feet on the bench. Press the dumb-bells up above your chest so that they are just touching each other. Your knuckles should be facing outwards.
Set yourself.

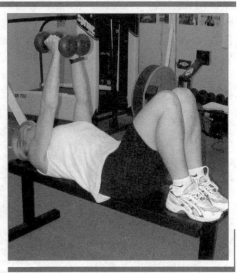

The exercise: To a count of 1-2-3 and while breathing in and with elbows slightly bent lower the dumb-bells to bench level, pause for 1 second, then to a count of 1-2 and while breathing out raise the dumb-bells with elbows still slightly bent, let the weights touch at the top of the press, pause for 1 second. Repeat.

Don't crash the dumb-bells together at the top of the press so that they bounce off each other.

Don't lower your arms below bench level.

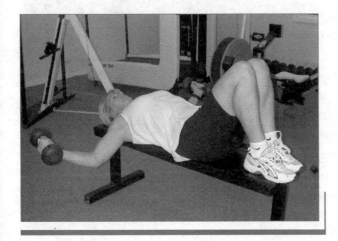

4. Barbell chest press (L2, L3)

Start: Lie flat on the bench with your feet on the bench. Grip the barbell slightly further apart than shoulder width and lift it off the uprights. Set yourself.

Don't attempt a barbell chest press with heavy weights without a 'spotter' (someone to help you).

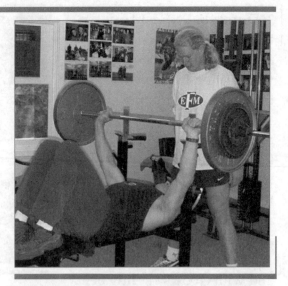

The exercise: Get a 'feel' of the weight before lowering to your mid-chest to a count of 1-2-3 while breathing in, pause for 1 second, then to a count of 1-2 and while breathing out press the weight up without locking out your elbows, pause for 1 second. Repeat.

Don't arch or lift your back while bench pressing and don't bounce the weight off your chest, because it's not necessary to get the barbell that low; you will achieve the desired results with this exercise by keeping your bent elbows parallel to the ground.

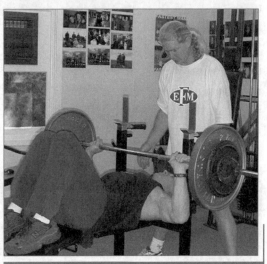

SHOULDERS

1. Dumb-bell seated shoulder press (PL1, L1, L2, L3)

Start: Hold the dumb-bells at shoulder level with knuckles facing towards you and with your feet comfortably apart. Set yourself.

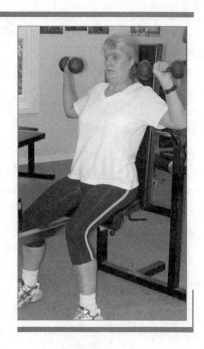

The exercise: To a count of 1-2 and while breathing out push the dumb-bells up and let them touch just above your head (at this point, your elbows are just slightly short of full extension), pause for 1 second, then to a count of 1-2-3 and while breathing in lower the dumb-bells to your starting position, pause for 1 second. Repeat.

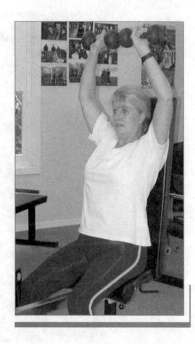

2. Dumb-bell standing shoulder lateral raise (L1, L2, L3)

Start: Hold the dumb-bells with your elbows at 90° and knuckles facing outwards.
Set yourself.

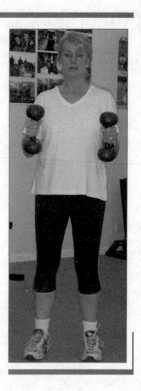

The exercise: To a count of 1-2 and while breathing out raise your elbows (still bent at 90°) to shoulder level, pause for 1 second, then to a count of 1-2-3 and while breathing in lower the dumb-bells to your starting position, pause for 1 second. Repeat.

NOTE that this exercise is preferred to side raises with straight elbows because it does the same job while reducing the risk of 'tennis elbow' and shoulder injury.

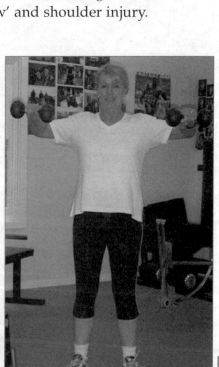

3. Barbell shoulder upright row (PL1, L1, L2, L3)

Start: Stand with legs at shoulder width, knees slightly bent and back braced. Hold the barbell at shoulder width and look straight ahead (maintain this head position through the exercise). Set yourself.

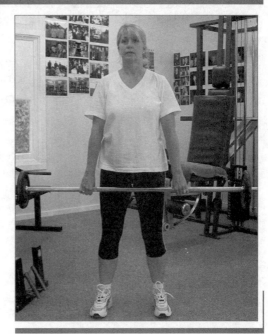

The exercise: To a count of 1-2 and while breathing out raise the barbell until your elbows reach shoulder height, pause for 1 second, then to a count of 1-2-3 and while breathing in lower the barbell to your starting position, pause for 1 second. Repeat.

Don't hold your hands close together.

Don't try to lift the barbell just under your chin.

Don't lean backwards.

NOTE that you can use dumb-bells to do this upright row.

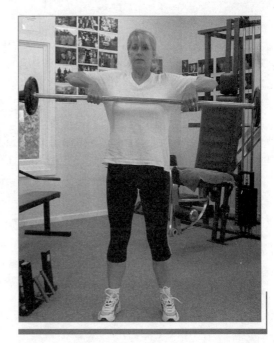

4. Dumb-bell shoulder front raise (L2, L3)

Start: Stand with knees slightly bent and your back firmly braced. Hold the dumb-bells on your thighs with knuckles facing away. Set yourself.

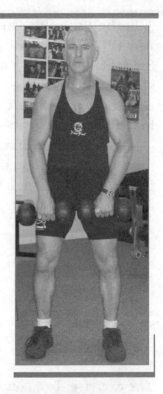

The exercise: With elbows slightly bent to a count of 1-2 and while breathing out raise your left arm to shoulder level, pause for 1 second, then to a count of 1-2-3 and while breathing in lower the weight to your starting position, pause for 1 second. Repeat on the other side.

NOTE that in this exercise the arms are raised alternatively. If you're doing 10 reps, this means 10 reps for each arm.

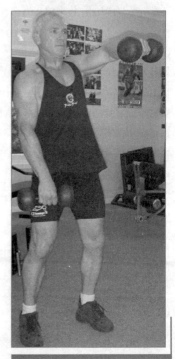

TRICEPS

1. Dumb-bell bent over triceps extension (PL1, L1, L2, L3)

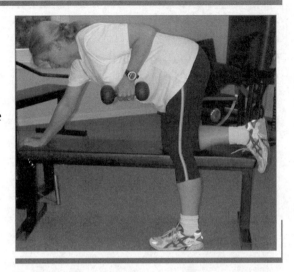

Start: Rest your right knee on the bench with your right arm extended and your elbow straight. You should be leaning forwards with your right arm supporting your upper body weight. Your left foot should be flat on the floor. Hold the dumb-bell in your left hand with the elbow flexed and elevated just above body level. Set yourself.

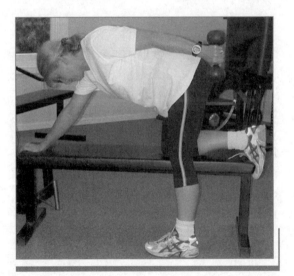

The exercise: To a count of 1-2 and while breathing out extend your elbow behind you, pause for 1 second, then to a count of 1-2-3 and while breathing in return to your starting position, pause for 1 second. Repeat. Complete your reps on this side before exercising the other side.

Don't allow the height of your elbow to fall or to rise. The key to this exercise is to hold your elbow at the same height while extending and flexing the elbow.

2. Dumb-bell seated triceps extension (L1, L2, L3)

Start: Hold the dumb-bell with both hands, palms facing upwards, and with the dumb-bell just below the back of your head. Set yourself.

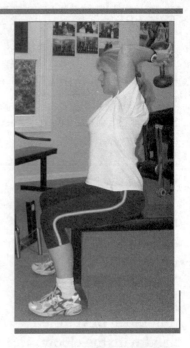

The exercise: To a count of 1-2 while breathing out raise the dumb-bell until your elbows are fully extended, pause for 1 second, then to a count of 1-2-3 and while breathing in lower the dumb-bell to your starting position, pause for 1 second. Repeat.

   Don't allow your elbows to splay out.

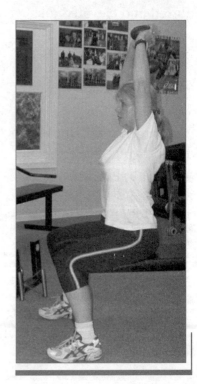

3. Cable triceps push down (PL1, L1, L2, L3)

Start: Stand with knees slightly bent and your back braced. Grip the T-bar with your knuckles facing upwards and your hands slightly narrower than shoulder width.
Set yourself.

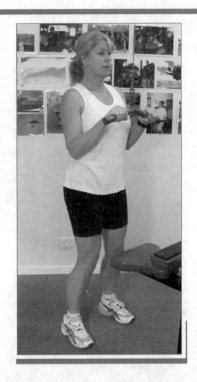

The exercise: To a count of 1-2 and while breathing out push the bar downwards towards your legs until your elbows are fully extended, pause for 1 second, then to a count of 1-2-3 and while breathing in allow the bar to return to your starting position, pause for 1 second. Repeat.

Don't let your elbows stray from their position next to your body.

Don't lean forwards or sideways so that your body weight forces the weight down.

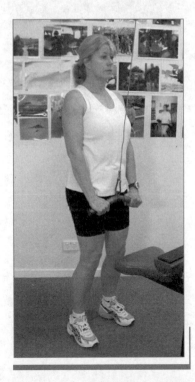

4. EZ bar triceps extension (L2, L3)
Start: Lie flat on the bench with your feet on the bench. Hold the EZ ('curly') bar or barbell with your hands just narrower than shoulder width and your elbows fully extended above you. Set yourself.

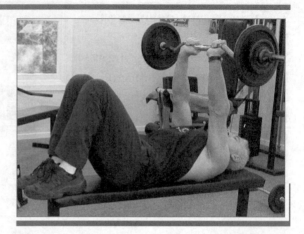

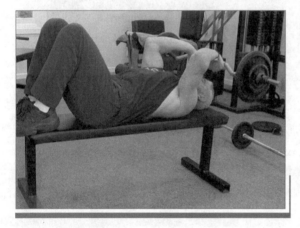

The exercise: To a count of 1-2-3 and while breathing in lower the weight to your forehead by bending the elbows, pause for 1 second, then to a count of 1-2 and while breathing out extend your elbows fully, pause for 1 second. Repeat.

Don't allow your elbows to move forwards.

BICEPS

1. Barbell standing biceps curls (L2, L3)

Start: Stand with your feet at shoulder width apart, knees slightly bent and back braced. Hold the barbell at shoulder width and with your elbows fully extended. Set yourself.

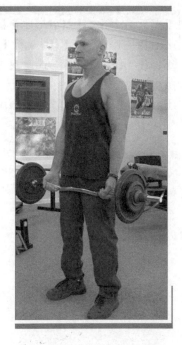

The exercise: Look straight ahead. To a count of 1-2 and while breathing out, fully flex your elbows, pause for 1 second, then to a count of 1-2-3 and while breathing in lower the barbell to your starting position, pause for 1 second. Repeat.

Don't lean backwards in order to lift the weight. In doing so, you not only avoid working the biceps properly, you also run the risk of back injury.

Don't keep your hands too close or too far apart; shoulder width is recommended.

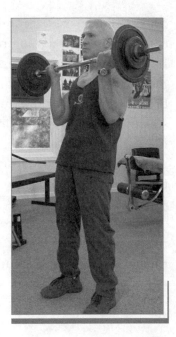

2. Dumb-bell standing biceps curls—no twist (PL1, L1, L2, L3)

Start: Stand with your feet shoulder width apart, your knees slightly bent and your back braced. Hold the dumb-bells on your thighs. Set yourself.

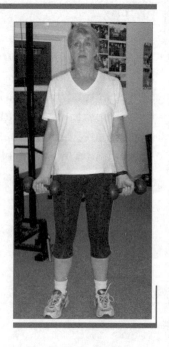

The exercise: Look straight ahead. To a count of 1-2 and while breathing out fully flex the right elbow, pause for 1 second, then to a count of 1-2-3 and while breathing in lower the dumb-bell to your starting position, pause for 1 second. Repeat on the other side.

Don't allow your elbows to stray from the side of your body.

Don't lean backwards.

NOTE that in this exercise the arms are raised alternately. If you are doing 10 reps this means 10 reps for each arm.

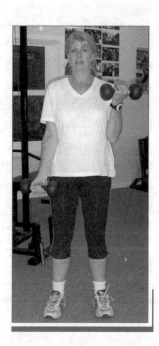

3. Dumb-bell seated biceps curls—with a twist (PL1, L1, L2, L3)

Start: Sit with your feet comfortably apart and your back (but not your head) firmly pressed against the backrest. Hold the dumb-bells with your elbows extended and your knuckles facing outwards.
Set yourself.

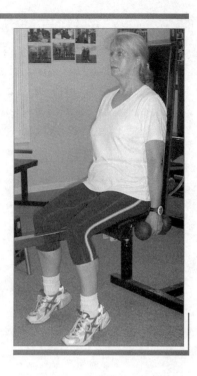

The exercise: To a count of 1-2 and while breathing out simultaneously rotate your left forearm and flex your elbow so that you finish up with your left elbow fully flexed and your knuckles facing away from you, pause for 1 second, then to a count of 1-2-3 and while breathing in lower the dumb-bell to your starting position, pause for 1 second. Repeat on the right side.

Don't throw your elbow outwards and rotate your body so that you get your shoulder under the lift.

Don't forget to concentrate on keeping your elbow close to your side.

NOTE that in this exercise the arms are raised alternately. If you're doing 10 reps, this means 10 reps for each arm.

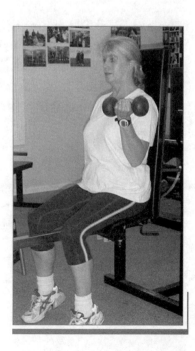

4. Dumb-bell standing biceps hammer curls (PL1, L1, L2, L3)

Start: Stand with your feet shoulder width apart, knees slightly bent and your back braced. Hold the dumb-bells by your sides, knuckles facing outwards. Set yourself.

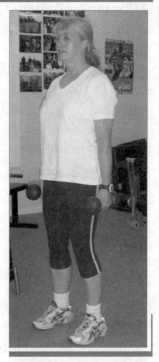

The exercise: To a count of 1-2 and while breathing out simultaneously flex both elbows keeping your knuckles facing outwards, pause for 1 second, then to a count of 1-2-3 and while breathing in lower the weights to your sides, pause for 1 second. Repeat.

Don't lean backwards.

Don't throw your elbows forward.

Don't extend the weights behind your body.

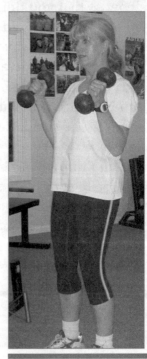

QUADRICEPS

1. Machine leg press (L2, L3)
Start: Irrespective of the sort of machine you are using it's terribly important to keep your back firmly braced against the back rest. This will reduce the risk of injury. Your feet should be shoulder width apart. Set yourself.

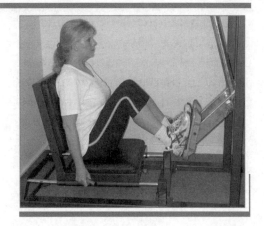

The exercise: Lower the weight slowly until your hips are flexed at 90° or at least to a point where you don't feel uncomfortable, then to a count of 1-2 and while breathing out push the weight away using your heels. It is important not to lock out your knees. Pause for 1 second, then to a count of 1-2-3 and while breathing in lower the weight, pause for 1 second. Repeat.

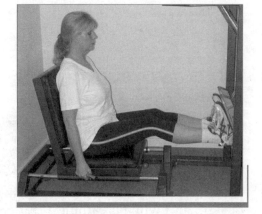

2. Machine quads extensions (PL1, L1, L2, L3)

Start: Make sure that your back is firmly pressed against the back rest of the leg extension machine and hold onto the side hand grips to give yourself stability. Set yourself.

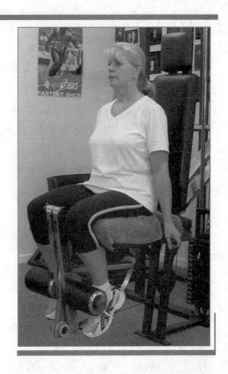

The exercise: To a count of 1-2 and while breathing out straighten your legs, pause for 1 second, then to a count of 1-2-3 and while breathing in lower the weight to your starting position, pause for 1 second. Repeat.

Don't do this exercise too fast.

Don't throw out your knees and allow them to return quickly to the start position, because this may result in injury.

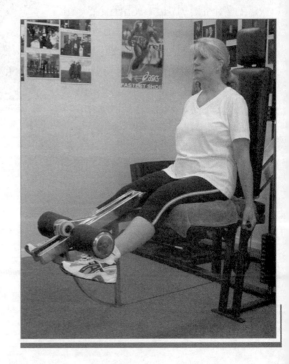

3. Fitness ball squats
(L1, L2, L3)

Start: Stand upright pressing the fitness ball against the wall with the small of your back (just above the buttocks) while holding the dumb-bells by your sides with your elbows extended.

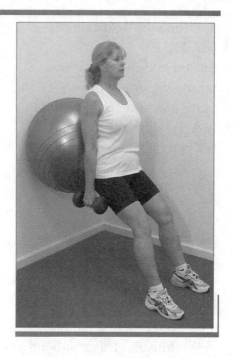

The exercise: To a count of 1-2-3 and while breathing in bend your knees to between 90° and 120° allowing the fitness ball to move up your back, pause for 1 second, and then to a count of 1-2 and while breathing out straighten your legs and return to the start position, pause for 1 second. Repeat.

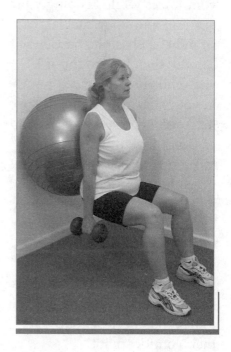

4. Dumb-bell squats
(L1, L2, L3)

Start: Hold the dumb-bells at your side with knuckles facing outwards and stand with your feet shoulder width apart.
Set yourself.

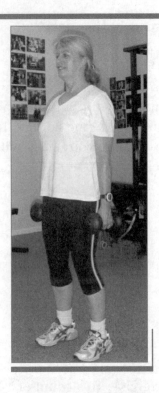

The exercise: To a count of 1-2-3 and while breathing in bend your knees while keeping your head up and your back as straight as possible, pause for 1 second, then to a count of 1-2 and while breathing out return to your starting position, pause for 1 second. Repeat.

Don't look down and *do* try to keep your back as straight as possible, because there is a natural tendency for it to bend.

NOTE that it's important to only flex your knees within your own capabilities. Older people and those with arthritis should not initially attempt to flex the knees beyond their comfort point.

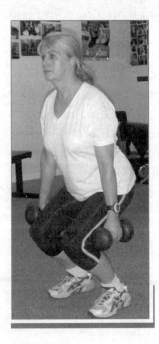

HAMSTRINGS

1. Machine hamstring curls (PL1, L1, L2, L3)

Start: Lie prone over the leg curl bench and hold the side grips for stability. Set yourself.

The exercise: To a count of 1-2 and while breathing out bend your knees as far as possible, pause for 1 second, then to a count of 1-2-3 and while breathing in lower the weight to your starting position, pause for 1 second. Repeat.

Don't use a weight that's too heavy, because it will encourage you to extend your back and this may lead to back strain.

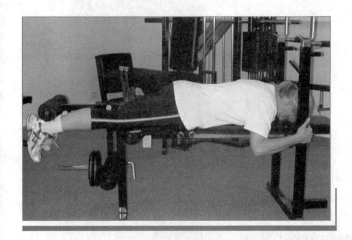

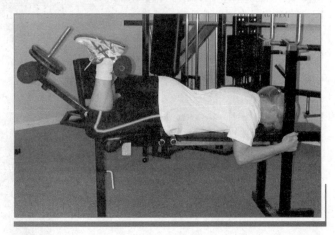

2. Dumb-bell lunges (L2, L3)

Start: Stand upright holding the dumb-bells with the knuckles facing outwards. Set yourself.

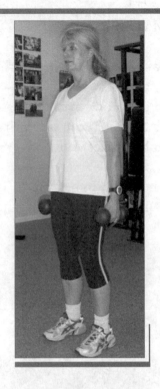

The exercise: Without moving your arms, step forward with your left foot allowing the left knee to bend and at the same time lowering your hips, then return to your starting position by pushing off with the left leg. Complete your full number of repetitions on your left leg, then switch to your right leg. Because of the nature of this exercise it's not possible to follow the 1-2, 1-2-3 rhythm.

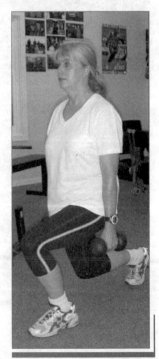

CALVES

1. Dumb-bell calf raises (PL1, L1, L2, L3)

Start: Hold the dumb-bell in your right hand with your right foot on the edge of a step and your right heel overhanging the step. Your left heel should be hooked behind your right leg and you should be holding onto a support with your left hand to maintain balance. Set yourself.

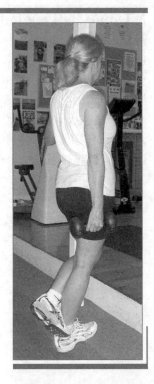

The exercise: To a count of 1-2 and while breathing out raise your right heel as far as you can, pause for 1 second, then to a count of 1-2-3 and while breathing in return to your starting position, pause for 1 second. Complete the repetitions on the right leg before moving to the left.

NOTE that it's important in this exercise that your calf moves in a straight line rather than outwards or inwards.

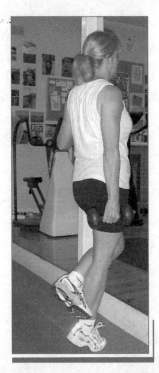

2. Dumb-bell angled calf raise
(PL1, L1, L2, L3)

Start: Stand with your legs shoulder width apart and your feet at a 45° angle. Hold a dumb-bell in each hand. Set yourself.

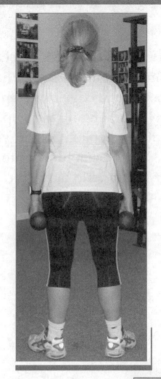

The exercise: To a count of 1-2 and while breathing out raise your heels as high as possible, pause for one second, then to a count of 1-2-3 and while breathing in lower your heels to the ground, pause for 1 second. Repeat.

Don't bend your knees while raising your heels.

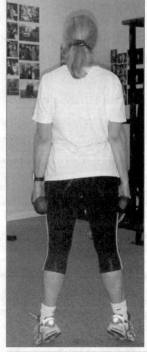

ABDOMINALS (ABS)

1. Upper ab crunches (PL1, L1, L2, L3)

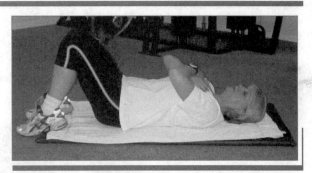

Start: Lie on a floor mat with your knees bent and your feet flat on the floor about 30 centimetres (1 foot) from your bottom. Cross your arms on your chest. Concentrate on flattening out (straightening) your lower back by imagining that you are pressing on a 20c piece—this requires a pelvic tilt (as in tilting your pubic bone towards your chin). This brings into play the lower part of the rectus abdominis muscle (a superficial abdominal muscle). At the same time you should pull your belly button up and backwards towards the spine, which brings into play the transversus abdominis muscle (a deep abdominal muscle, see Chapter 17).

The exercise: While breathing out begin your crunch by bringing your shoulders off the mat until your shoulder blades are about to leave the mat, pause at the 'crunch' before slowly returning to your starting position.

NOTE that it's important throughout this exercise to maintain the downward pressure on the imaginary 20c piece. As you get stronger with this exercise you can use a starting position with your shoulders off the mat and crunch upwards before returning to the same position. You'll find that your range of movement with this crunch exercise is very small because it isolates the abdominal muscles' movement.

2. Lower abs crunches (PL1, L1, L2, L3)

This is identical to the previous exercise (upper ab crunches) except that it's performed with your ankles crossed and your feet just off the floor, where they remain throughout the duration of the exercise.

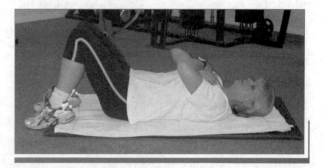

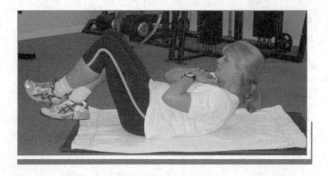

3. Fitness ball crunches
(PL1, L1, L2, L3)

Start: Lie on the fitness ball with your feet shoulder width apart and with the ball sitting comfortably in your lower back. Keep your backside firmly pressed against the ball throughout the exercise. Cross your arms over your chest. Set yourself.

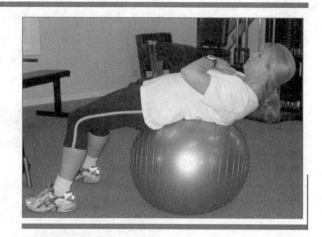

The exercise: To a count of 1-2 and while breathing out raise your trunk while crunching down, pause for 1 second, then to a count of 1-2-3 and while breathing in lower your trunk to your starting position, pause for 1 second. Repeat.

Don't bring your trunk up to a sitting position when doing the sit-up, because you'll lose the 'crunch'.

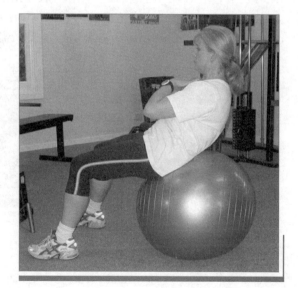

4. Side crunches (PL1, L1, L2, L3)

Start: Lie flat on your back with your knees bent on the left side. Place your left hand on the left side of your chest and cover it with your right hand. Set yourself.

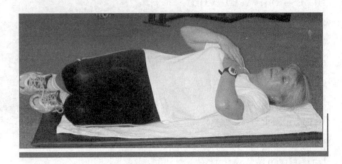

The exercise: To a count of 1-2 and while breathing out raise your upper body towards your right hip, pause for 1 second, then to a count of 1-2-3 and while breathing in return to your starting position, pause for 1 second. Complete your repetitions on the right side before switching to the other side.

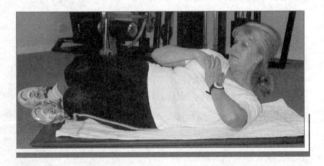

BACK EXTENSION EXERCISES

1. Back paddle
(PL1, L1, L2, L3)
Start: Lie prone with arms and legs extended. It often helps to place a rolled-up towel between your belly button and hips.
Set yourself.

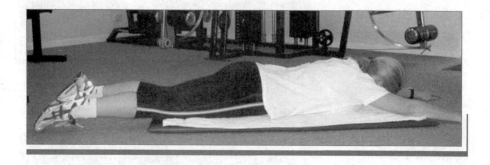

The exercise: Simultaneously raise your right arm and left leg as far as you can, then lower them to the floor. Repeat on the other side.

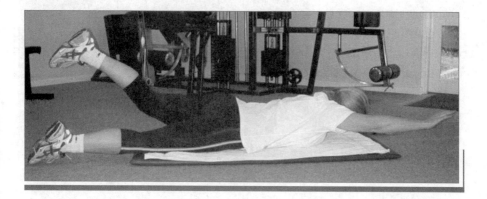

2. Fitness ball back extensions (PL1, L1, L2, L3)

Start: Kneel in front of the fitness ball with your ~~knees~~ *thighs* just touching the ball and with your hands at the back of your head. Set yourself.

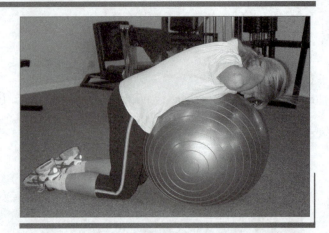

The exercise: To a count of 1-2 and while breathing out raise your trunk off the ball as far as you can, pause for 1 second, then to a count of 1-2-3 and while breathing in lower your trunk onto the ball, pause for 1 second. Repeat.

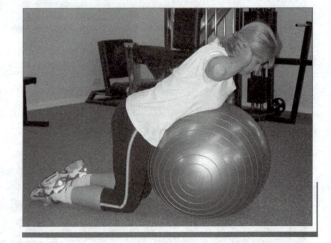

RESISTANCE BANDS EXERCISES

Resistance bands are graded in strength of elasticity and are colour coded. Special handles can be purchased with resistance bands and are useful for some of the exercises. You'll need a 1 metre (about 3 foot) length of band for your routine.

Resistance bands are useful for people with arthritis and for older adults. They provide resistance throughout the range of movement, and the slower the movement the greater resistance. Some of you may start with resistance bands and later move on to free weights or weight machines. If you intend to stick with resistance bands only, it will be necessary to have two or three bands of different strengths. Resistance bands are inexpensive and have the advantage of being easily transportable.

It is just as important to follow the principles of resistance training (discussed in Chapter 10) when using resistance bands as it is with free weights or weight machines. It is particularly important to control the band using a 1-2 rhythm on the lifting (power) phase and a 1-2-3 rhythm on the lowering (relaxation) phase. Always keep your wrists firm and in a neutral position (i.e. neither flexed nor extended).

An important point in resistance band exercises is to set or stabilise yourself before each set of exercises. If you fail to do this you may unnecessarily load the supporting ('facet') joints in your lower back (lumbar) area and you will place load on your ligaments. Not only can this lead to injury, but it means you will not get as much out of the exercise because your upper body (trunk) has not been stabilised.

Remember the 'PS'—position and stability (see Chapter 10). Now you're stabilised and ready to go!

LATS/BACK

1. Resistance band lats pull-down (PL1, L1)

Start: Cross the band over a horizontal bar (e.g. a railing). Grip one part of the band in each hand with your arms at 100°–120°. Set yourself and keep your wrists firm.

The exercise: To a count of 1-2 and while breathing out pull the bands to your outer thighs, pause for 1 second, then to a count of 1-2-3 and while breathing in allow the band to return to your starting position. Repeat.

NOTE that the band has some degree of stretch throughout this exercise.

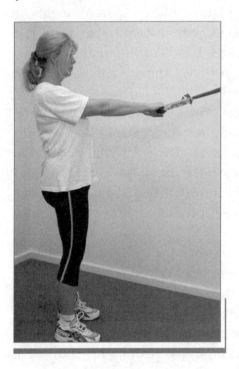

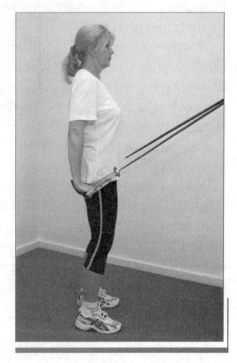

2. Resistance band lats/back seated row (PL1, L1)

Start: Sit on the floor with legs straight out in front and with the band passing under the instep of your shoes. Grip one part of the band in each hand.
Set yourself and keep your wrists firm.

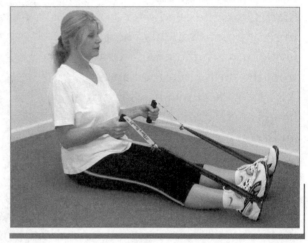

The exercise: To a count of 1-2 and while breathing out pull your hands level to your chest, pause for 1 second, then to a count of 1-2-3 and while breathing in allow the bands to return to your start position. Repeat.

NOTE that you'll probably need to hold the band short at the start of the exercise. The band has some degree of stretch throughout this exercise.

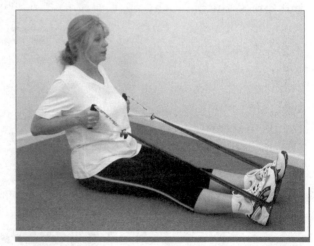

CHEST

1. Resistance band standing chest press (PL1, L1)

Start: Cross the band over an upright post at roughly chest level. Turn around and face away from the post. Hold the hands with knuckles upwards and with hands at chest level. Set yourself and keep your wrists firm.

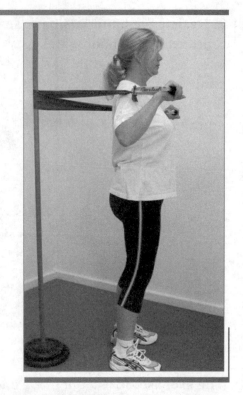

The exercise: To a count of 1-2 and while breathing out 'press' the bands away from you, keeping your arms at chest level, pause for 1 second, then to a count of 1-2-3 and while breathing in allow the bands to return to your starting position. Repeat.

Don't allow your body to sway forward, because then your body weight and not your chest muscles will be doing the work.

NOTE that the band has some degree of stretch throughout this exercise.

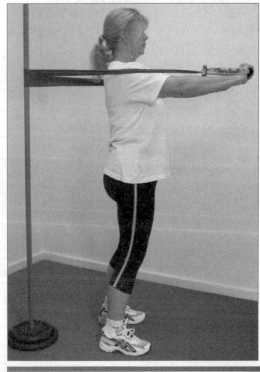

2. Resistance band seated chest press (PL1, L1)

Start: Cross the bands over the back of a chair at roughly chest level. Turn around and sit down. Hold the handles with knuckles upwards and with hands at chest level. Set yourself and keep your wrists firm.

The exercise: To a count of 1-2 and while breathing out 'press' the bands away from you keeping your arms at chest level, pause for 1 second then to a count of 1-2-3 and while breathing in allow the bands to return to your starting position.

NOTE that the band is on some degree of stretch throughout this exercise (it may be necessary to hold the band short to get sufficient tension).

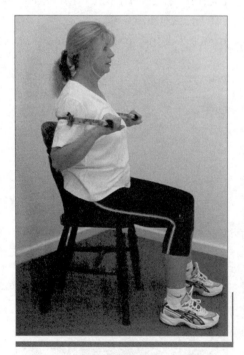
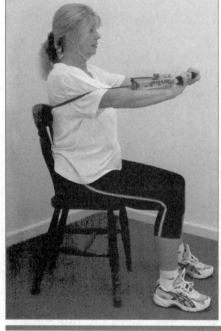

SHOULDERS

1. Resistance band shoulder 'skiing' (PL1, L1)

Start: Stand on the band with feet shoulder width apart. The knuckles should be facing forwards and your arms at your side.

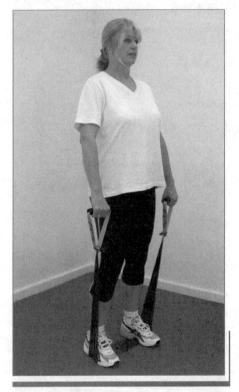

The exercise: To a count of 1-2 and while breathing out bring your right arm forward to no more than 60° while simultaneously moving your left arm back to no more than 30°. Then to a count of

1-2 and while breathing in repeat the process on the other side. You should complete your 'breathing in' phase when your arms pass your body.

Don't bend your elbows. This exercise works the anterior and the posterior parts of the deltoid muscle and will only do so if you keep your elbows straight.

NOTE that this is quite a rhythmic exercise. The rhythm is therefore faster than with most other resistance exercises—hence 1-2 'in' and 1-2 'out'.

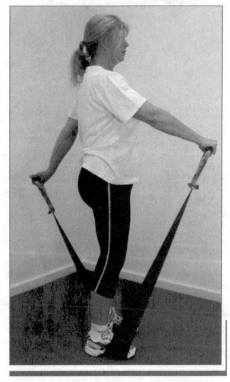

2. Resistance band shoulder internal rotation (PL1, L1)

Start: Tie one end of the band to an upright pole. Hold the handle in your right hand, knuckles facing the pole and with your right elbow fixed at 90°. Set yourself with your wrist firm. Make certain that in the start position the band is taut.

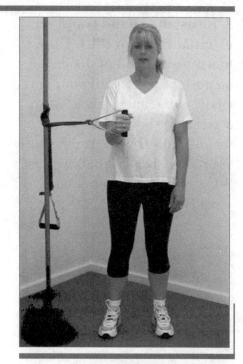

The exercise: To a count of 1-2 and while breathing out move your right arm across your upper abdomen, pause for 1 second, then to a count of 1-2-3 and while breathing in allow the band to return to your starting position. Complete your set and then repeat on the other side.

Don't allow your elbow to move away from your side.

NOTE that at the start of the exercise the band must be sufficiently taut so that there is always tension on it during both the lifting (power) phase and lowering (relaxation) phase of the exercise.

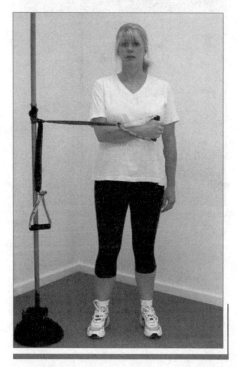

3. Resistance band shoulder external rotation (PL1, L1)

Start: Tie one end of the band to an upright pole. With your left elbow at 90° and your left arm across your body, grab onto the handle of the band. At this point your knuckle is facing the pole. Set yourself and keep your wrist firm.

The exercise: To a count of 1-2 and while breathing out move your left arm away from your abdomen until it will go no further, pause for 1 second, then to a count of 1-2-3 and while breathing out allow your left arm to return to its starting position. Complete your set and then repeat on the other side.

Don't allow your left elbow to move away from your side.

NOTE that the band is on some degree of stretch throughout this exercise.

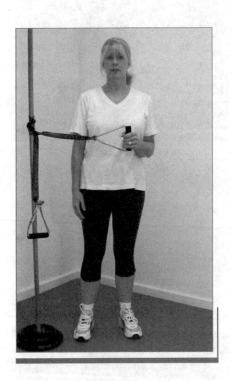

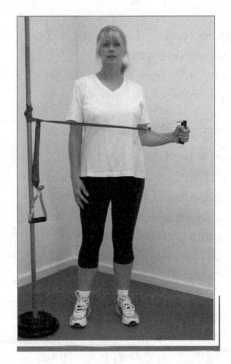

TRICEPS

1. Resistance band standing triceps extension (PL1, L1)

Start: Tie one end of the band to an upright pole. While facing the pole, hold the handle with your knuckles facing upwards and your elbow bent at 90°. Set yourself and keep your wrist firm.

The exercise: To a count of 1-2 and while breathing out extend your elbow (at the completion of which your elbow should be straight alongside your body), pause for 1 second, then to a count of 1-2-3 and while breathing in allow your arm to return to its starting position. Complete your set and then repeat on the other side.

Don't allow your elbow to move away from the side of your body.

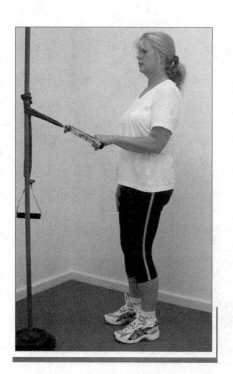
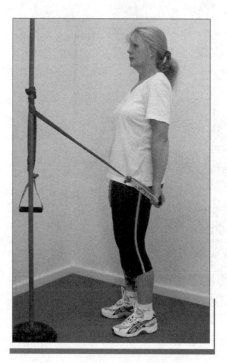

BICEPS

1. Resistance band standing biceps curl (PL1, L1)

Start: Stand on the band with your feet shoulder width apart. Hold the handles in each hand with your knuckles facing backwards and your arms fully extended by your sides. Set yourself and keep your wrists firm.

The exercise: To a count of 1-2 and while breathing out bend your elbows as far as they will go, pause for 1 second, then to a count of 1-2-3 and while breathing in allow your arms to return to their starting position. Repeat.

Don't allow your elbows to move away from the sides of your body.

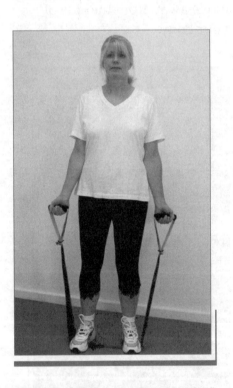

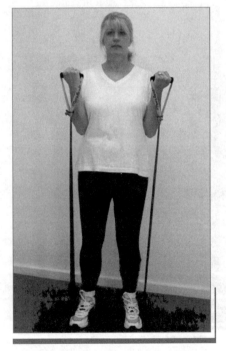

QUADRICEPS

1. Resistance band seated quads extension (PL1, L1)

Start: Sit on a chair (the higher the better). Tie one end of the band to the chair leg (tie it short so that there is tension in the band). Place your foot in the handle. Set yourself and hold onto the sides of the chair to provide stability.

The exercise: To a count of 1-2 and while breathing out extend your right knee (to 90° if you can), pause for 1 second, then to a count of 1-2-3 and while breathing in allow your leg to return to its starting position. Complete your set and repeat on the other side.

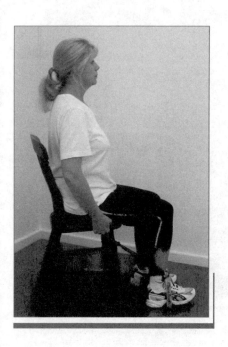

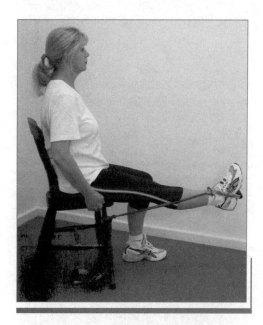

2.Resistance band quads squats (PL1, L1)

Start: Stand on the band with feet at shoulder width apart. Hold the handles in each hand with your knuckles facing outwards. In this exercise the band needs to be on a fairly tight stretch in the three-quarter knee bent position. Set yourself and keep your wrists firm.

The exercise: To a count of 1-2 and while breathing out straighten your knees and hips so that you are standing upright, pause for 1 second, then to a count of 1-2-3 and while breathing in return to your three-quarter knee bent starting position. Repeat.

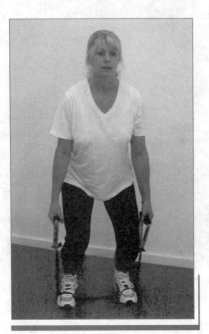
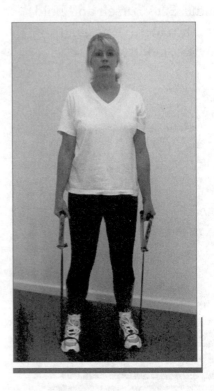

HAMSTRINGS

1. Resistance band standing hamstring flexion (PL1, L1)

Start: Tie one end of the band to an upright pole. Place your left foot in the handle. Keep your right knee pressing against your left and hold on to the upright pole for balance. Set yourself.

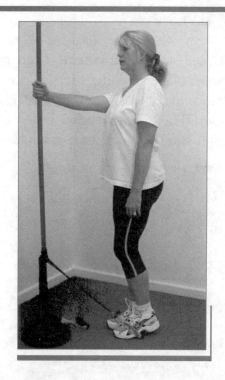

The exercise: To a count of 1-2 and while breathing out bend your left knee as far as it will go, pause for 1 second, then to a count of 1-2-3 and while breathing in allow your foot to return to your starting position. Complete your set and repeat on the other side.

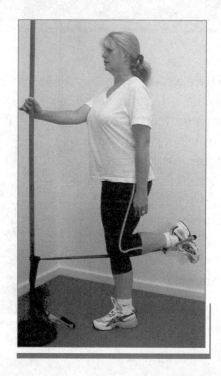

CALVES

1. Resistance band seated calf raise (PL1, L1)

Start: Place your right foot in the handle of the band and hold the band under tension with your right hand behind you. Your knee should be fully extended and your foot drawn up as far as it will go towards your knee. Set yourself.

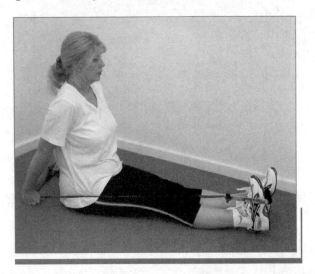

The exercise: To a count of 1-2 and while breathing out move your foot downwards, pause for 1 second, then to a count of 1-2-3 and while breathing in draw your foot towards you. Complete your set and then repeat on the other side.

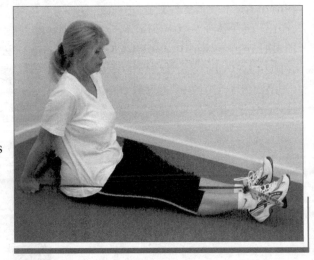

Chapter 13 Resistance training levels

| 'Singlemindedness is
| all powerful.'

YAMAMOTO TSUNETOMO,
THE BOOK OF THE SAMURAI (HAGAKURE)

Before deciding the resistance training level at which you should start your program, it is first necessary to determine the weight you should be lifting. First-time weight exercisers should be conservative and err on the side of beginning with light weights. Do this and you'll experience less muscle soreness. You will still make progress and within a short time will probably want to go on to a higher weight. Always keep in mind the principles we discussed in Chapter 10, namely the importance of not lifting a weight so heavy that it compromises good form, body position and stability, or lifting rhythm.

HOW TO DETERMINE YOUR LIFTING WEIGHT FOR RESISTANCE TRAINING

Step 1. Do your 'stretch-up' as shown in Chapter 11.

Step 2. Lift the heaviest weight you can lift once. This will vary from muscle group to muscle group. Larger muscles are the stronger. For example, the quadriceps (thigh muscles) are the largest in the body and you'll be able to lift roughly three or four times more weight in a machine quads extension than in a biceps exercise.

Step 3. The weight you lift when training will be somewhere between 60% and 80% of the heaviest weight you can lift once.

When first lifting a weight which is 60–80% of your maximum you may feel it's too light, but remember this is a training weight. You won't be lifting this weight only once in your resistance training program. You may be doing up to 12 reps per set of a particular exercise and you'll be doing a number of sets. You will see that in Pre-Level 1 (low intensity), Level 1 (low intensity) and Level 2 (moderate intensity) the recommended training weight is less than 80% of your maximum single lift. However, if you are older your maximum lift may not be very much, so that even 80% of this weight may provide only moderate resistance. In this case, stick with 80%. Using only a modest weight in the beginning is often helpful until you've learned the correct form of the exercise. You can then move on to a weight sufficient to provide the amount of 'overload' to build muscle and strength.

When attempting your maximum single lift you should do so under the supervision of a fitness instructor. If the instructor has any concerns about your health or your capacity to attempt a maximum single lift, then he or she may advise that you postpone this until after a preparatory conditioning period with light weights.

HOW TO DETERMINE YOUR STARTING LEVEL FOR RESISTANCE TRAINING

The level at which you start your resistance training program is not determined by how much weight you can lift. You may have a lot of natural strength and be capable of lifting a big weight, but if you haven't previously trained with weights then your supporting and anchoring tissues (ligaments and tendons) will not be conditioned for training with weights. Unconditioned supporting tissues are prone to injury—especially as we get older. It won't matter how strong your muscles are if the tendons attaching the muscles to the bone are a weak link. In the 40-plus age group common 'weak links' are the tendons that attach muscle to the elbow. Injury to these tendons can lead to 'tennis elbow' and 'golfer's elbow'. The rotator cuff of the shoulder is also a weak link—an injury to this can lead to 'tendinitis'. Another weak link is the wrist, which is why it's so important to keep it 'locked' when exercising—especially when using resistance bands.

If you've had little if any prior conditioning with weights, don't let your natural strength tempt you into starting at too high a level. If you're at all doubtful at which level you should begin, err on the side of caution. You can always go up to the next level a little sooner, and I can tell you that's a lot better than having to go down a level because of injury.

IDENTIFYING THE LEVEL FOR YOU
Pre-Level 1 (low intensity)
This is recommended:

- For the 60–90 year old age group, particularly if you've never previously done any regular exercise (resistance or cardiovascular), and for those who may have previously exercised but some time ago.
- For those with severe arthritis (Functional Class 3 and some in Functional Class 2—see Chapter 7)
- Your training weight should be 60% of your maximum single lift.

If your grip strength is such that you can't lift weights (e.g. hand deformities caused by arthritis), then it's recommended that you use resistance bands (see Chapter 12). If you feel you're in the Pre-Level 1 category and will be able to work only with resistance bands, I recommend that you determine your personal resistance band strength with the assistance of a trained instructor or physiotherapist. If using free weights, then for the first two weeks you may find it helpful to use low weights while you familiarise yourself with the exercises. Another helpful strategy is to initially only do very low reps (no more than 5). This will avoid muscle soreness, which older adults may find interferes with their daily activities.

Level 1 (low intensity)

This is recommended:

- For those under 60 years who may have never previously done any regular exercise (resistance or cardiovascular) and for those who may have last exercised only some time ago.
- For those with mild to moderate arthritis.
- Your training weight should be 60–65% of your maximum single lift.

Level 2 (moderate intensity)

This is recommended:

- For those who've been doing some form of regular exercise, be this resistance training or cardiovascular training. This may include some people with mild arthritis who've been regular exercisers.
- Your training weight should be 70–75% of your maximum single lift.

Level 3 (high intensity)

This is recommended:

- For those who are currently weight training. If you've had past experience with weight training but haven't done any for a while, it's recommended that you make a start at Level 2, even if for only 6 weeks, before moving on to Level 3.
- Your training weight should be 80% of your maximum single lift.

At Level 3 you should be looking for challenges and variations. Many people involved in regular resistance training fall into the trap (or habit) of following the same exercise pattern week after week. In time, the exercises become easier and easier because muscles adapt to the same routine. Not only does this lead to boredom, but your strength is likely to plateau because your muscles are no longer being challenged ('overloaded'). This can lead to staleness, which is often misinterpreted as overtraining. For this reason I've recommended that at Level 3, two different training patterns be used and rotated every three to four weeks. For convenience I've called these Training Pattern A (TPA) and Training Pattern B (TPB).

Chapter 14   Resistance training programs

> *'Everyone lets the present
> moment slip by,
> and looks for it as though
> he thought it was
> somewhere else.'*

YAMAMOTO TSUNETOMO,
THE BOOK OF THE SAMURAI (HAGAKURE)

TRAINING PROGRAM FOR LEVEL 1 (LOW INTENSITY)

This program for Level 1 is also suitable for those Pre-Level 1 exercisers who are able to use free weights or machines. However, it is important that you use weights that are not too heavy (be this 60% or 80% of your single maximum lift) and you should do only half the reps recommended for Level 1. If you can't use free weights you'll find at the end of this chapter a special Pre-Level 1 program using resistance bands.

WEEKS 1–3
Day 1 (Monday)
(1) *Stretch-up.*
(2) *Plan:* upper body workout—all main muscle groups starting with the largest: lats/back followed by chest, shoulders, triceps and biceps; two different abs exercises.
(3) *Strategy:*
    (i) Choose one Level 1 exercise per body part from Chapter 12 (note that each exercise in Chapter 12 has a code next to it indicating the level it's suitable for, i.e. PL1, L1, L2, L3). Write

down on your workout sheet what exercises you've done and, if you like, note how you felt (too easy, not quite hard enough, too hard, etc.).

(ii) Do two sets of 10 reps per exercise with a 1 minute break between sets.

(iii) Have a $1^1/2$ minute break after the second set of each exercise before moving on to the next exercise.

(iv) Once you've completed your upper body workout, do two different abs exercises. Do one set of 15 reps for each of the two abs exercises you've chosen, with a 1 minute break between sets.

(4) *Stretch-down.*

Your workout sheet will look something like this (as mentioned earlier, pounds are common in gyms so I've given them here; 1 kilogram is 2.2 lb).

Exercise	*Kg*	Weight	Reps	Break
Cable lats pull down	*18*	40 lb	10	1 min
		40 lb	10	$1^1/2$ min
Dumb-bell chest press	*7*	15 lb	10	1 min
		15 lb	10	$1^1/2$ min
Dumb-bell seated shoulder press	*4.5*	10 lb	10	1 min
		10 lb	10	$1^1/2$ min
Dumb-bell bent-over triceps ext		10 lb	10	1 min
		10 lb	10	$1^1/2$ min
Dumb-bell standing biceps curls— no twist		10 lb	10	1 min
		10 lb	10	$1^1/2$ min
Upper abs crunches			15	1 min
Lower abs crunches			15	0 min

The whole workout, including stretching up and stretching down, should take no more than 30 minutes.

Day 2 (Wednesday)

(1) *Stretch-up.*

(2) *Plan*: upper body workout—all main muscle groups starting with the largest, just as we did on Day 1; two different abs exercises.

(3) *Strategy*:

    (i) Choose one Level 1 exercise per body part from Chapter 12 but make it a different exercise for that body part from the exercise you did on Day 1; write down on your workout sheet what exercises you've done and how you felt.

    (ii) Do two sets of 10 reps per exercise with a 1 minute break between sets.

    (iii) Have a $1^1/2$ minute break after the second set of each exercise before moving on to the next exercise.

    (iv) Once you've completed your upper body workout do two different abs exercises. Do one set of 15 reps for each of the two abs exercises you've chosen, with a 1 minute break between sets.

(4) *Stretch-down.*

Your workout sheet will look something like this.

Exercise	Weight	Reps	Break
Cable reverse grip lats pull down	40 lb	10	1 min
	40 lb	10	$1^1/2$ min
Dumb-bell incline chest press	15 lb	10	1 min
	15 lb	10	$1^1/2$ min
Dumb-bell standing shoulder lateral raise	10 lb	10	1 min
	10 lb	10	$1^1/2$ min
Dumb-bell seated triceps ext	15 lb	10	1 min
	15 lb	10	$1^1/2$ min
Dumb-bell seated biceps curls—twist	10 lb	10	1 min
	10 lb	10	$1^1/2$ min
Fitness ball crunches		15	1 min
Side crunches		15	0 min

(Handwritten annotations in the Kg column: 18, 7, 4.5, 7, 4.5)

The whole workout including stretching up and stretching down should take no more than 30 minutes.

Day 3 (Friday)

(1) *Stretch-up.*

(2) *Plan*: lower body workout—all main muscle groups starting with the largest, quadriceps, followed by hamstrings followed by calves; three different abs exercises; two different back extension exercises.

(3) *Strategy*:

    (i) Choose one Level 1 exercise per body part from Chapter 12; write down on your workout sheet what exercises you've done and how you felt.

    (ii) Do three sets of 10 reps per exercise, with a 1 minute break between sets.

    (iii) Have a 2 minute break after the third set of each exercise before moving on to the next exercise.

    (iv) Once you've completed your lower body workout do three different abs exercises. Do one set of 15 reps for each of the three abs exercises you've chosen, with a 1 minute break between sets.

    (v) Do one set of 15 reps for each of the two back extension exercises you've chosen, with a 1 minute break between sets.

(4) *Stretch-down.*

Your workout sheet will look something like this.

Exercise	*Kg*	Weight	Reps	Break
Machine quads ext		30 lb	10	1 min
	13·5	30 lb	10	1 min
		30 lb	10	2 min
Machine hamstring curls		15 lb	10	1 min
	7	15 lb	10	1 min
		15 lb	10	2 min
Dumb-bell calf raises		15 lb	10	1 min
		15 lb	10	1 min
		15 lb	10	2 min
Lower abs crunches			15	1 min

Exercise	Weight	Reps	Break
Fitness ball crunches		15	1 min
Side crunches		15 (each side)	1 min
Back paddles		15 (each side)	1 min
Fitness ball back ext		15	0 min

The whole workout, including stretching up and stretching down, should take no more than 30 minutes.

You've just completed Week 1 of Level 1. You've achieved your first mini-goal. You're on your way. Continue the pattern through Weeks 2 and 3 but don't be afraid of making use of different exercises from Chapter 12 for the same body part. This provides variation and makes for more interesting workouts. Note that you're doing two upper body workouts and one lower body workout. The reason for this is that on one or two days of the week when you're not doing resistance training you should be undertaking cardiovascular exercise, which will also work your legs; this will be covered in Chapter 15.

WEEKS 4–6
Day 1 (Monday)
(1) *Stretch-up.*

(2) *Plan*: upper body workout—all main muscle groups starting with the largest; two different abs exercises.

(3) *Strategy*:
   (i)   Choose one Level 1 exercise per body part from Chapter 12; write down on your workout sheet what exercises you've done and how you felt.

   (ii) Do three sets of 10 reps per exercise, with a 1 minute break between sets.

   (iii) Have a $1^1/2$ minute break after the third set of each exercise before moving on to the next exercise.

   (iv) Once you've completed your upper body workout do two different abs exercises. Do one set of 15 reps for each of the two abs exercises you've chosen, with a 1 minute break between sets. Keep the weights for upper body exercises the same as in Weeks 1–3, because remember you're now doing an extra set.

(4) *Stretch-down.*

Your workout sheet will look something like this.

Exercise	Kg	Weight	Reps	Break
Cable lats pull down		40 lb	10	1 min
	18	40 lb	10	1 min
		40 lb	10	1½ min
Dumb-bell chest press		15 lb	10	1 min
	7	15 lb	10	1 min
		15 lb	10	1½ min
Dumb-bell seated		10 lb	10	1 min
shoulder press	4·5	10 lb	10	1 min
		10 lb	10	1½ min
Dumb-bell bent-over		10 lb	10	1 min
triceps ext		10 lb	10	1 min
		10 lb	10	1½ min
Dumb-bell standing biceps curls—		10 lb	10	1 min
no twist		10 lb	10	1 min
		10 lb	10	1½ min
Upper abs crunches			15	1 min
Lower abs crunches			15	0 min

The whole workout, including stretching up and stretching down, may take 30–40 minutes.

Day 2 (Wednesday)
(1) *Stretch-up.*

(2) *Plan*: upper body workout—all main muscle groups starting with the largest; do two different abs exercises.

(3) *Strategy*:

    (i) Choose one Level 1 exercise per body part from Chapter 12 but make it a different exercise for that body part from the exercise you did on Day 1; write down on your workout sheet what exercises you've done and how you felt.

    (ii) Do three sets of 10 reps per exercise, with a 1 minute break between sets.

    (iii) Have a 1^1/$_2$ minute break after the third set of each exercise before moving on to the next exercise.

    (iv) Once you've completed your upper body part workout do two different abs exercises. Do one set of 15 reps for each of the two abs exercises you've chosen, with a 1 minute break between sets.

(4) *Stretch-down.*

Your workout sheet will look something like this.

Exercise	Weight	Reps	Break
Cable reverse grip lats pull-down	40 lb	10	1 min
	40 lb	10	1 min
	40 lb	10	1½ min
Dumb-bell incline chest press	15 lb	10	1 min
	15 lb	10	1 min
	15 lb	10	1½ min
Dumb-bell standing shoulder lateral raise	10 lb	10	1 min
	10 lb	10	1 min
	10 lb	10	1½ min

Exercise	Kg	Weight	Reps	Break
Dumb-bell seated		15 lb	10	1 min
triceps ext	7	15 lb	10	1 min
		15 lb	10	1½ min
Dumb-bell seated biceps		10 lb	10	1 min
curls—twist	4·5	10 lb	10	1 min
		10 lb	10	1½ min
Fitness ball crunches			15	1 min
Side crunches			15 (each side)	0 min

The whole workout, including stretching up and stretching down, should take around 40 minutes.

Day 3 (Friday)

(1) *Stretch-up.*

(2) *Plan*: lower body workout—all main muscle groups starting with the largest, quadriceps, followed by hamstrings followed by calves; three different abs exercises; two different back extension exercises.

(3) *Strategy*:

(i) Choose one Level 1 exercise per body part from Chapter 12; write down on your workout sheet what exercises you've done and how you felt.

(ii) Do three sets of 10 reps per exercise with a 1 minute break between sets but increase the weight by 5 lb.

(iii) Have a 2 minute break after the third set of each exercise before moving onto the next exercise.

(iv) Once you've completed your lower body workout do three different abs exercises. Do one set of 15 reps for each of the three abs exercises you've chosen, with a 1 minute break between sets.

(v) Do one set of 15 reps for each of the two back extension
       exercises you've chosen, with a 1 minute break between sets.

(4) *Stretch-down.*

Your workout sheet will look something like this.

Exercise	*Kg*	Weight	Reps	Break
Machine quads ext		35 lb	10	1 min
	16	35 lb	10	1 min
		35 lb	10	2 min
Machine hamstring curls		20 lb	10	1 min
	9	20 lb	10	1 min
		20 lb	10	2 min
Dumb-bell calf raises		20 lb	10	1 min
		20 lb	10	1 min
		20 lb	10	2 min
Lower abs crunches			15	1 min
Side crunches			15 (each side)	1 min
Back paddles			15 (each side)	1 min
Fitness ball back ext			15	0 min

The whole workout, including stretching up and stretching down,
should take around 35 minutes.

TRAINING PROGRAM FOR LEVEL 2 (MODERATE INTENSITY)

WEEKS 1–6
Day 1 (Monday)

(1) *Stretch-up.*

(2) *Plan*: upper body workout—all main muscle groups starting with
    the largest; two different abs exercises.

(3) *Strategy*:

(i) Choose one Level 2 exercise per body part from Chapter 12;

write down on your workout sheet what exercises you've
done and how you felt.

(ii) Do three sets of 10 reps per exercise, with a 1 minute break
between sets.

(iii) Have a 2 minute break after the third set of each exercise
before moving on to the next exercise.

(iv) Once you've completed your upper body workout do
two different abs exercises. Do one set of 25 reps for each
of the two abs exercises you have chosen, with a 1 minute
break between sets.

(4) *Stretch-down*.

Your workout sheet will look something like this.

Exercise	*Kg*	Weight	Reps	Break
Cable lats pull down		50 lb	10	1 min
	23	50 lb	10	1 min
		50 lb	10	2 min
Dumb-bell chest press		25 lb	10	1 min
	11·5	25 lb	10	1 min
		25 lb	10	2 min
Dumb-bell seated		20 lb	10	1 min
shoulder press	*9*	20 lb	10	1 min
		20 lb	10	2 min
Dumb-bell bent-over		15 lb	10	1 min
triceps ext	*7*	15 lb	10	1 min
		15 lb	10	2 min
Dumb-bell standing biceps curls—		15 lb	10	1 min
no twist		15 lb	10	1 min
		15 lb	10	2 min
Upper abs crunches			25	1 min
Lower abs crunches			25	0 min

The whole workout, including stretching up and stretching down,
should take around 45 minutes.

Day 2 (Wednesday)

(1) *Stretch-up.*

(2) *Plan*: upper body workout—all main muscle groups starting with the largest; two different abs exercises.

(3) *Strategy*:

    (i) Choose one Level 2 exercise per body part from Chapter 12 but make it a different exercise for that body part from the exercise you did on Day 1; write down on your workout sheet what exercises you've done and how you felt.

    (ii) Do three sets of 10 reps per exercise, with a 1 minute break between sets.

    (iii) Have a 2 minute break after the third set of each exercise before moving on to the next exercise.

    (iv) Once you've completed your upper body workout do two different abs exercises. Do one set of 30 reps for each of the two abs exercises you have chosen, with a 1 minute break between sets.

(4) *Stretch-down.*

Your workout sheet will look something like this.

Exercise	Weight	Reps	Break
Dumb-bell one arm lats row	30 lb	10	1 min
	30 lb	10	1 min
	30 lb	10	2 min
Dumb-bell incline chest press	25 lb	10	1 min
	25 lb	10	1 min
	25 lb	10	2 min
Dumb-bell standing shoulder lateral raise	15 lb	10	1 min
	15 lb	10	1 min
	15 lb	10	2 min

(Handwritten annotations: "Kg", "13·5" next to lats row, "11·5" next to chest press, "7" next to shoulder raise.)

Exercise	Kg	Weight	Reps	Break
Cable triceps push-down		30 lb	10	1 min
	13·5	30 lb	10	1 min
		30 lb	10	2 min
Dumb-bell seated biceps-		20 lb	10	1 min
curls—twist	*9*	20 lb	10	1 min
		20 lb	10	2 min
Fitness ball crunches			30	1 min
Side crunches			30 (each side)	0 min

The whole workout, including stretching up and stretching down, should take around 45 minutes.

Day 3 (Friday)
(1) *Stretch-up*.
(2) *Plan*: lower body workout—all main muscle groups starting with the largest; three different abs exercises; two different back extension exercises.
(3) *Strategy*:
   (i) Choose two Level 2 exercises per body part from Chapter 12; write down on your workout sheet what exercises you've done and how you felt.
   (ii) Do three sets of 10 reps per exercise, with a 1 minute break between sets.
   (iii) Have a 2 minute break after the third set of each exercise before moving on to the next exercise.
   (iv) Once you've completed your lower body workout, do three different abs exercises. Do one set of 30 reps for each

of the three abs exercises you have chosen, with a 1 minute break between sets.

(v) Do one set of 20 reps for each of the two back extension exercises you have chosen, with a 1 minute break between sets.

(4) *Stretch-down.*

Your workout sheet will look something like this.

Exercise	*Kg*	Weight	Reps	Break
Machine leg press		100 lb	10	1 min
	45·5	100 lb	10	1 min
		100 lb	10	2 min
Machine quads ext		40 lb	10	1 min
	18	40 lb	10	1 min
		40 lb	10	2 min
Machine hamstring curls		25 lb	10	1 min
	11·5	25 lb	10	1 min
		25 lb	10	2 min
Dumb-bell lunges		20 lb	10	1 min
	9	20 lb	10	1 min
		20 lb	10	2 min
Dumb-bell calf raises		30 lb	10	1 min
	13·5	30 lb	10	1 min
		30 lb	10	2 min
Dumb-bell angled calf raises		25 lb	10	1 min
	11·5	25 lb	10	1 min
		25 lb	10	2 min
Lower abs crunches			30	1 min
Fitness ball crunches			30	1 min
Side crunches			30 (each side)	1 min
Back paddles			20 (each side)	1 min
Fitness ball back ext			20	0 min

The whole workout, including stretching up and stretching down, should take no more than 45 minutes.

TRAINING PROGRAM FOR LEVEL 3 (HIGH INTENSITY)

WEEKS 1–3—TRAINING PATTERN A (TPA)
Day 1 (Monday) & Day 2 (Wednesday)
(1) *Stretch-up.*
(2) *Plan:* upper body workout—all main muscle groups starting with the largest; two different abs exercises.
(3) *Strategy:*
   (i) Choose two Level 3 exercises per body part from Chapter 12; write down on your workout sheet what exercises you've done and how you felt.
   (ii) Do three sets of 10 reps per exercise, with a 1 minute break between sets.
   (iii) Have a 2 minute break after the third set of each exercise before moving on to the next exercise.
   (iv) Once you've completed your upper body workout do two different abs exercises. Do one set of 50 reps (or more) for each of the two abs exercises that you have chosen, with a 1 minute break between sets.
(4) *Stretch-down.*

Your workout sheet will look something like this.

Exercise	*Kg*	Weight	Reps	Break
Cable lats pull down		150 lb	10	1 min
	68	150 lb	10	1 min
		150 lb	10	2 min
Dumb-bell one arm lats row		80 lb	10	1 min
	36·5	80 lb	10	1 min
		80 lb	10	2 min
Barbell chest press		176 lb (80 kg)	10	1 min
	80	176 lb	10	1 min
		176 lb	10	2 min

Exercise	*Kg*	Weight	Reps	Break
Dumb-bell chest flys	*23*	50 lb	10	1 min
		50 lb	10	1 min
		50 lb	10	2 min
Dumb-bell seated shoulder press	*18*	40 lb	10	1 min
		40 lb	10	1 min
		40 lb	10	2 min
Dumb-bell shoulder front raise	*13.5*	30 lb	10	1 min
		30 lb	10	1 min
		30 lb	10	2 min
Cable triceps pushdown	*27.5*	60 lb	10	1 min
		60 lb	10	1 min
		60 lb	10	2 min
EZ Bar triceps ext	*40*	88 lb (40 kg)	10	1 min
		88 lb	10	1 min
		88 lb	10	2 min
Barbell standing biceps curls		88 lb (40 kg)	10	1 min
		88 lb	10	1 min
		88 lb	10	2 min
Dumb-bell seated biceps curls—twist	*16*	35 lb	10	1 min
		35 lb	10	1 min
		35 lb	10	2 min
Fitness ball crunches			100	1 min
Side crunches			50	0 min

The whole workout, including stretching up and stretching down, should take 50–60 minutes.

Day 3 (Friday)

(1) *Stretch-up.*

(2) *Plan:* lower body workout—all main muscle groups starting with the largest; three different abs exercises; two different back extension exercises.

(3) *Strategy:*

(i) Choose two Level 3 exercises per body part from Chapter 12; write down on your workout sheet what exercises you've done and how you felt.

(ii) Do three sets of 10 reps per exercise, with a 1 minute break between sets.

(iii) Have a 2 minute break after the third set of each exercise before moving on to the next body part.

(iv) Once you've completed your lower body workout do three different abs exercises. Do one set of at least 50 reps for each of the three abs exercises you've chosen, with a 1 minute break between sets.

(v) Do one set of 20 reps for each of the two back extension exercises you've chosen, with a 1 minute break between sets.

(4) *Stretch-down.*

Your workout sheet will look something like this.

Exercise	*Kg*	Weight	Reps	Break
Machine leg press	*68*	150 lb	10	1 min
		150 lb	10	1 min
		150 lb	10	2 min
Machine quads ext	*36·5*	80 lb	10	1 min
		80 lb	10	1 min
		80 lb	10	2 min
Machine hamstring curls	*18*	40 lb	10	1 min
		40 lb	10	1 min
		40 lb	10	2 min

Exercise	*Kg*	Weight	Reps	Break
Dumb-bell lunges		30 lb	10	1 min
	13·5	30 lb	10	1 min
		30 lb	10	2 min
Dumb-bell calf raises		50 lb	10	1 min
	23	50 lb	10	1 min
		50 lb	10	2 min
Dumb-bell angled calf raises		40 lb	10	1 min
	18	40 lb	10	1 min
		40 lb	10	2 min
Upper abs crunches			50	1 min
Lower abs crunches			50	1 min
Fitness ball crunches			50	0 min
Back paddles			20 (each side)	1 min
Fitness ball back ext			20	0 min

The whole workout, including stretching up and stretching down, should take 40–45 minutes.

WEEKS 4–6—TRAINING PATTERN B (TPB)

Day 1 (Monday) & Day 2 (Wednesday)

(1) *Stretch-up*.

(2) *Plan*: upper body workout—all main muscle groups starting with the largest; two different abs exercises.

(3) *Strategy*:

  (i)   Choose one Level 3 exercise per body part from Chapter 12; write down on your exercise sheet what exercises you've done and how you felt.

  (ii) 'Pyramid' six sets per body part, working 'bottom to top—top to bottom': reps: 12-9-6-6-9-12 with a 1 minute break between sets. Note how the weight is increased over the first three sets, the fourth set is done at the same weight as the third set before reducing to the starting weight (see workout sheet below).

(iii) Have a 2 minute break after the sixth set before moving on to the next exercise.

(iv) Once you've completed your upper body workout do two different abs exercises. Do one set of at least 50 reps for each of the two abs exercises you've chosen, with a 1 minute break between sets.

(4) *Stretch-down.*

Your workout sheet will look something like this.

Exercise	Kg	Weight	Reps	Break
Cable reverse grip lat pull-down	50	110 lb	12	1 min
	59	130 lb	9	1 min
	68	150 lb	6	1 min
		150 lb	6	1 min
	59	130 lb	9	1 min
	50	110 lb	12	2 min
Dumb-bell incline chest press	18	40 lb	12	1 min
	20·5	45 lb	9	1 min
	25	55 lb	6	1 min
		55 lb	6	1 min
	20·5	45 lb	9	1 min
	18	40 lb	12	2 min
Dumb-bell shoulder front raise	11·5	25 lb	12	1 min
	13·5	30 lb	9	1 min
	16	35 lb	6	1 min
		35 lb	6	1 min
	13·5	30 lb	9	1 min
	11·5	25 lb	12	2 min

Exercise	Kg	Weight	Reps	Break
EZ bar triceps ext	*27.5*	60 lb	12	1 min
	32	70 lb	9	1 min
	36.5	80 lb	6	1 min
		80 lb	6	1 min
	32	70 lb	9	1 min
	27.5	60 lb	12	2 min
Dumb-bell seated biceps curls—twist	*13.5*	30 lb	12	1 min
	16	35 lb	9	1 min
	18	40 lb	6	1 min
		40 lb	6	1 min
	16	35 lb	9	1 min
	13.5	30 lb	12	2 min
Fitness ball crunches			100	1 min
Upper abs crunches			50	0 min

The whole workout, including stretching up and stretching down, should take 50–60 minutes.

Day 3 (Friday)
(1) *Stretch-up.*
(2) *Plan*: lower body workout—all main muscle groups starting with the largest; three different abs exercises; two different back extension exercises.
(3) *Strategy*:
    (i) Choose one Level 3 exercise per body part from Chapter 12; write down on your workout sheet what exercise you've done and how you felt.
    (ii) Pyramid sets per body part, working 'bottom to top—top to bottom'; reps: 12-9-6-6-9-12 with a 1 minute break between sets.
    (iii) Have a 2 minute break after the sixth set before moving on to the next exercise.

(iv) Once you've completed your lower body workout do three different abs exercises. Do one set of at least 50 reps for each of the three abs exercises you have chosen with a 1 minute break between sets.

(v) Do one set of 25 reps for each of the two back extension exercises you've chosen, with a 1 minute break between sets.

(4) *Stretch-down.*

Your workout sheet will look something like this.

Exercise	*Kg*	Weight	Reps	Break
Machine quads ext	*27·5*	60 lb	12	1 min
	32	70 lb	9	1 min
	36·5	80 lb	6	1 min
		80 lb	6	1 min
	32	70 lb	9	1 min
	27·5	60 lb	12	2 min
Machine hamstring curls	*13·5*	30 lb	12	1 min
	18	40 lb	9	1 min
	23	50 lb	6	1 min
		50 lb	6	1 min
	18	40 lb	9	1 min
	13·5	30 lb	12	2 min
Dumb-bell calf raises	*18*	40 lb	12	1 min
	23	50 lb	9	1 min
	27·5	60 lb	6	1 min
		60 lb	6	1 min
	23	50 lb	9	1 min
	18	40 lb	12	2 min
Upper abs crunches			50	1 min
Lower abs crunches			50	1 min
Fitness ball crunches			50	1 min
Back paddles			25	1 min
Fitness ball back ext			25	0 min

The whole workout, including stretching up and stretching down, should take 45–50 minutes.

After completing this 4–6 weeks period of TPB, return to TPA for 1 to 3 weeks and then repeat TPB and so on.

As you become more experienced at Level 3 you can develop further routines. You may want to do some concentrated muscle building by focusing on only two muscle groups/body parts per training session, e.g. chest/biceps or back/triceps or shoulders/biceps or some other suitable combination. In this case you can do three different exercises per muscle group/body part and do three sets of 10 reps per exercise or you can do two pyramid sets for each of the body parts.

TRAINING PROGRAM FOR PRE-LEVEL 1 (LOW INTENSITY) USING RESISTANCE BANDS

(Suitable for people who cannot use free weights or weight machines)

WEEKS 1–6
Day 1 (Monday) & Day 2 (Wednesday)

(1) *Stretch-up.*

(2) *Plan*: upper body workout—all main muscle groups starting with the largest; lats/back, followed by chest, shoulders, triceps, biceps; two different abs exercises.

(3) *Strategy*:

  (i)   Choose one resistance band exercise per body part from Chapter 12; write down on your workout sheet what exercises you've done and how you felt.

  (ii) Do two sets of 10 reps per exercise, with a 1 minute break between sets.

  (iii) Have a $1^1/2$ minute break after the second set of each exercise before moving on to the next exercise.

  (iv) Once you've completed your upper body workout do two different abs exercises. Do one set of 15 reps for each of

the two abs exercises you've chosen, with a 1 minute
break between sets.
(4) *Stretch-down.*

Your workout sheet will look something like this.

Exercise	Reps	Break
Resistance band lats pull down	10	1 min
	10	1½ min
Resistance band standing	10	1 min
chest press	10	1½ min
Resistance band shoulder 'skiing'	30 (total)	1 min
	30 (total)	1½ min
Resistance band standing triceps ext	10	1 min
	10	1½ min
Resistance band standing biceps curl	10	1 min
	10	1½ min
Upper abs crunches	15	1 min
Lower abs crunches	15	0 min

The whole workout, including stretching up and stretching down,
should take no more than 30 minutes.

Day 3 (Friday)
(1) *Stretch-up.*
(2) *Plan*: lower body workout—all main muscle groups starting with
the largest: quads followed by hamstrings, followed by calves;
three different abs exercises; two different back extension exercises.
(3) *Strategy*:
    (i) Choose one resistance band exercise from Chapter 12; write
down on your workout sheet what exercise you've done and
how you felt.

(ii) Do three sets of 10 reps per exercise, with a 1 minute break between sets.

(iii) Have a 2 minute break after the third set of each exercise before moving on to the next exercise.

(iv) Once you've completed your lower body workout do three different abs exercises. Do one set of 15 reps for each of the three abs exercises you've chosen, with a 1 minute break between sets.

(v) Do one set of 15 reps for each of the two back extension exercises you've chosen, with a 1 minute break between sets.

(4) *Stretch-down*.

Your workout sheet will look something like this.

Exercise	Reps	Break
Resistance band quads seated ext	10	1 min
	10	1 min
	10	2 min
Resistance band standing hamstring flex	10	1 min
	10	1 min
	10	2 min
Resistance band seated calf raise	10	1 min
	10	1 min
	10	2 min
Lower abs crunches	15	1 min
Fitness ball crunches	15	1 min
Side crunches	15 (each side)	1 min
Back paddles	15 (each side)	1 min
Fitness ball back ext	15	0 min

The whole workout, including stretching up and stretching down, should take no more than 30 minutes.

WEEKS 7–12
Day 1 (Monday) & Day 2 (Wednesday)
(1) *Stretch-up.*
(2) *Plan*: upper body workout—all main muscle groups starting with the two largest; two different abs exercises.
(3) *Strategy*:
   (i) Choose one resistance band exercise from Chapter 12 but try to make it a different exercise for that body part from the exercise you did in weeks 1–6. Write down on your workout sheet what exercises you've done and how you felt.
   (ii) Do three sets of 10 reps per exercise, with a 1 minute break between sets.
   (iii) Have a $1^1/_2$ minute break after the third set of each exercise before moving on to the next exercise.
   (iv) Once you've completed your upper body workout do two different abs exercises. Do one set of 15 reps for each of the two abs exercises you've chosen, with a 1 minute break between sets.
(4) *Stretch-down.*

Your workout sheet will look something like this.

Exercise	Reps	Break
Resistance band lats pull down	10	1 min
	10	1 min
	10	$1^1/_2$ min
Resistance band seated chest press	10	1 min
	10	1 min
	10	$1^1/_2$ min
Resistance band shoulder int rotation	10 (each side)	1 min
	10 (each side)	1 min
	10 (each side)	$1^1/_2$ min
Resistance band standing triceps ext	10	1 min
	10	1 min
	10	$1^1/_2$ min

Exercise	Reps	Break
Resistance band standing biceps curl	10	1 min
	10	1 min
	10	1½ min
Upper abs crunches	15	1 min
Lower abs crunches	15	0 min

The whole workout, including stretching up and stretching down, should take no more than 30 minutes.

Day 3 (Friday)

(1) *Stretch-up*.

(2) *Plan*: lower body workout—all main muscle groups starting with the largest: quads followed by hamstrings followed by calves; three different abs exercises; two different back extension exercises.

(3) *Strategy*:

    (i) Choose one resistance band exercise per body part from Chapter 12; write down on your workout sheet what exercise you've chosen and how you felt.

    (ii) Do three sets of 20 reps per exercise, with a 1 minute break between sets.

    (iii) Have a 2 minute break after the third set of each exercise before moving on to the next exercise.

    (iv) Once you've completed your lower body workout do three different abs exercises. Do one set of 25 reps (or more) for each of the three abs exercises you've chosen, with a 1 minute break between sets.

    (v) Do one set of 20 reps for each of the two back extension exercises you've chosen, with a 1 minute break between sets.

(4) *Stretch-down*.

Your workout sheet will look something like this.

Exercise	Reps	Break
Resistance band quads squats	20	1 min
	20	1 min
	20	1½ min
Resistance band standing hamstring flexion	20	1 min
	20	1 min
	20	1½ min
Resistance band seated calf raise	20	1 min
	20	1 min
	20	1½ min
Lower abs crunches	25	1 min
Fitness ball crunches	25	1 min
Side crunches	25 (each side)	1 min
Back paddles	20 (each side)	1 min
Fitness ball back ext	20	0 min

The whole workout, including stretching up and stretching down, should take no more than 40 minutes.

IMPORTANT NOTE FOR PRE-LEVEL 1 EXERCISES

If at any stage you feel that Pre-Level 1 resistance band exercises are not sufficiently challenging then you should move to Level 1.

If you feel you are unable to use free weights but would still like to increase the intensity of your resistance band workouts, then you'll need to use a resistance band with a higher degree of tension or alternatively increase your reps.

WHEN TIME IS OF THE ESSENCE

It will sometimes happen that despite your best intentions and your best-laid plans there's just no way you can get to the gym.

Something's come up. An important work or social engagement, an obligation you're bound to keep—your training schedule is history. The good thing is you know all of this in advance. You can't get to the gym but you've got 30 minutes at home to do something. In fact, all the time you'll need to do a modified workout. All you need is one set of dumb-bells—anything between 5 pounds and 25 pounds, depending on your strength and fitness. If you happen to be in the vicinity of a set of dumb-bells that you feel are too light for you then do what I call the 'TITE' (Time Is of The Essence) workout with 30 reps per set. It's quick, it's fast, you'll sweat and it works. Do the reps quickly rather than using the 1-2: 1-2-3 cadence, but remember to breathe out when lifting the weight and to breathe in when lowering it. Afterwards make certain that you drink enough water—you'll need it.

THE TITE WORKOUT (HIGH INTENSITY)

Your workout sheet will look something like this.

Exercise	Reps	Break
SHOULDERS		
1. Dumb-bell standing shoulder press	15	30 sec
	15	30 sec
	15	30 sec
2. Dumb-bell shoulder standing front raise	15	30 sec
	15	30 sec
	15	30 sec
3. Dumb-bell standing upright row	15	30 sec
	15	30 sec
	15	30 sec
TRICEPS		
4. Dumb-bell bent over triceps ext	15	30 sec
(if you don't have a bench	15	30 sec
use a box or a stool)	15	30 sec

Exercise	Reps	Break
5. Dumb-bell seated triceps ext	15	30 sec
	15	30 sec
	15	30 sec
6. Push-ups (with hands shoulder	15	30 sec
width apart)	15	30 sec
	15	30 sec
BICEPS		
7. Dumb-bell standing curls	15	30 sec
(no twist *and* with both arms together)	15	30 sec
	15	30 sec
8. Dumb-bell standing	15	30 sec
hammer curls	15	30 sec
(both arms together)	15	30 sec
ABS		
9. Upper abs crunches	50	30 sec
10. Lower abs crunches	50	30 sec
11. Side crunches	25	30 sec
	25	0 sec

Chapter 15

Cardiovascular training

| *'Life is an endurance test, so why be ashamed of your age.'*

P.K. SHAW

CARDIOVASCULAR TALK

Aerobic: literally means 'with oxygen'. It describes how our body, and in particular our muscles, are working most of the time. The opposite of aerobic is 'anaerobic' which means 'without oxygen'.

Our muscles simply cannot function without oxygen for too long. As a matter of fact, they're designed not to do so! If our muscles are deprived of oxygen for too long they very rapidly accumulate hydrogen ions (like lactic acid) that interfere with the muscles' ability to keep on contracting. No matter how strong-willed you might be, if too many hydrogen ions accumulate, your muscles will seize up and stop working. Of course most of us are unlikely to ever have such an experience. It's the sort of thing that may happen to highly trained athletes at the end of a 400 metre race (which is really a prolonged sprint). You may sometimes see such athletes collapsing to the ground at the end of a race. Spectators often think that the athlete is just throwing himself across the finishing line but in fact his muscles have simply seized up because of the high build-up of hydrogen ions. This is sometimes referred to as 'oxygen debt'. The way the muscles 'pay back' the debt is by going on strike! They temporarily stop working. The prime purpose for doing so is to protect the muscles against permanent damage that would otherwise occur were the muscles able to continue functioning for a prolonged period without oxygen. Of course the athlete who collapses will rapidly recover normal function once the oxygen debt is paid back. Herein lies an important message. It's virtually impossible to permanently damage muscle through 'overuse'. The one exception to this is a situation in which a person who is grossly dehydrated continues to exercise for a prolonged period at extremely high temperatures. This may result in the rare condition of 'muscle melt-down'. There is no likelihood of this occurring in a gym situation. In fact, the more you use a muscle the stronger it becomes, making it less liable to injury.

Cardiovascular: the 'cardio' part of this term refers to the heart and the 'vascular' part refers to the blood vessels. Thus, 'cardiovascular' simply means heart and vessels. The term 'cardiovascular training' is used to describe the sort of training that increases the efficiency of heart *and* lung function ('cardiorespiratory' would really be more accurate, since 'respiratory' refers to the lungs, but let's not be picky). Cardiovascular training is also described as 'endurance training'. You'll find that the terms 'cardiovascular training', 'endurance training' and 'aerobic training' are often used interchangeably. The American College of Sports Medicine defines cardiovascular exercise as any mode of continuous activity using large muscle groups that is rhythmic and aerobic in nature. However there may be certain times during cardiovascular training (e.g. when doing Level 3 interval training) when you are working anaerobically, so that not all 'cardiovascular training' is necessarily purely aerobic. This is why I prefer the term 'cardiovascular training' to 'aerobic training'.

WHY COMBINE CARDIOVASCULAR TRAINING AND RESISTANCE TRAINING?
BENEFITS OF CARDIOVASCULAR TRAINING
Earlier on we discussed how resistance training can build muscle and reduce body fat, and in this way enhance the ability to undertake cardiovascular exercise more efficiently. It also works the other way. By having cardiovascular fitness your ability (endurance) to undertake resistance exercises will be enhanced. Resistance training and cardiovascular training should be seen as working together.

Some of the benefits that we described in Chapter 8 resulting from resistance training will also occur with cardiovascular training. However cardiovascular training won't give you the same improvements in muscle mass, strength or metabolic rate, nor will it significantly prevent or reduce the risk of osteoporosis unless the cardiovascular training is of the 'high-impact aerobic' variety, which is considered unsuitable for many older adults and people with arthritis. This is why we combine resistance training with low-impact cardiovascular training. This will achieve exactly the same level of cardiovascular fitness as high-impact aerobics without putting older and/or arthritic joints at risk

Weight reduction and reducing the risks of diabetes and osteoarthritis

Cardiovascular training is a great way to burn kilojoules. Because you have increased your muscle mass and reduced your body fat with resistance training you'll now burn kilojoules even more efficiently. This will help weight reduction, thereby reducing the risk of diabetes and the likelihood of developing osteoarthritis of the weight-bearing joints. If you already have arthritis in your leg joints, weight reduction will help to reduce the pain of arthritis.

Reduction in cardiovascular disease (heart attack, stroke) and high blood pressure

When you exercise, your muscles need and in fact demand more oxygen. Your heart meets these demands by beating faster. Remember, your heart too is made of muscle (a special kind of muscle but nevertheless muscle). By having to beat faster and pump more blood to meet the increased demands of your arm and leg muscles while you are training, you are also training your heart muscle (the 'cardio' part of cardiovascular training). Your heart will get bigger and the blood vessels that supply the heart muscle actually grow to accommodate the growth of your heart muscle. Now, because your heart is a more efficient pump it doesn't have to work as hard to pump out the same amount of blood. Instead of having to pump say 84 times a minute to get the blood to circulate around your body, it may now need to pump only 60 times a minute or even less. This is why fit athletes have very low resting heart rates. You will too. Chances are that because your heart doesn't have to work as hard to get its job done, it may keep working for longer.

We know that cardiovascular training lowers 'bad' (LDL) cholesterol and increases 'good' (HDL) cholesterol. That's good too because it reduces the risk of plaques forming in your arteries and thereby reduces the risk of heart disease, stroke and high blood pressure.

Increased endurance

Cardiovascular training increases the efficiency of function of your heart, lungs and muscles, which results in increased endurance. We call this *cardiovascular fitness*. Studies have shown that increased endurance in the elderly following cardiovascular training is similar to that reported in middle-aged and younger adults. Furthermore, responses to training are not affected by gender, or by menopause. Greater endurance means less fatigue, and an ability to accomplish more in your day.

Sense of well-being

Cardiovascular fitness is associated with high levels of endorphins— chemicals in the body that give us a sense of well-being, improve pain tolerance and reduce depression and anxiety.

MAXIMUM HEART RATE

Your maximum heart rate will be age-dependent. A simple way to calculate your maximum heart rate is to take away from the number 220 your age in years. If you are 50 years old then your maximum heart rate will be 170 (220 − 50). Of course there will be individual variations. Another way of determining maximum heart rate is by a 'symptom-limited' exercise stress test. This involves walking or running on a treadmill until a point is reached where you can no longer continue to participate in the activity. In most cases this will simply be the result of exhaustion, but people with coronary artery disease may be forced to stop the activity because of chest pain (angina). Whether or not the activity is ceased because of exhaustion or chest pain, it is at that point that the heart rate is measured. This is your maximum heart rate. These tests are costly and time consuming. They are recommended only for people who are considered to have risk factors for heart disease or a known history of heart disease.

You can monitor your own heart rate very easily during exercise simply by taking your pulse. Of course you will momentarily have to stop whatever exercise you are doing in order to do this.

How to take your pulse

With the palm of your right hand facing upwards and the right wrist bent slightly back, place your left index and middle fingers on the thumb-side of your right wrist. It is not necessary to press too hard. Count the number of beats for 15 seconds and multiply by 4. This will give you your heart rate in beats per minute. I recommend the use of a heart rate monitor for over-40 exercisers—as much for safety as for actually monitoring your exercise intensity level. They are available at most sports shops. They consist of a thin rubber strap which is worn around the lower chest and a wrist watch which provides a display of your heart rate. These cost around A$99.00 for the simplest model and are an excellent and convenient way to monitor your exercise intensity.

EXERCISE INTENSITY

It is important to realise that the benefits of cardiovascular training are 'dose related' and will depend on the quality (intensity) and quantity (frequency and duration) of exercise. However, just moving from a sedentary lifestyle to even a minimal level of physical activity will deliver significant health benefits. Programs that involve a higher training intensity and more frequent training sessions will provide additional benefits. To obtain a meaningful increase in cardiovascular fitness (endurance) requires a minimum of two cardiovascular training sessions of moderate intensity per week. If you have a low (or very low) level of fitness then initially you'll be able to train at only a low intensity (see below). In this case you should train more frequently (four or five times a week) and your training duration will need to be longer (40 to 60 minutes). *This need not be continuous.* You can achieve the same result by accumulating a number of shorter sessions (minimum 10 minutes) throughout the day. If you have a moderate to high level of fitness or attain this through training then, because you will be able to train at a higher intensity, your training duration can be shorter (20 to 30 minutes).

LOW-INTENSITY EXERCISE (Pre-Level 1 and Level 1)

This describes exercise which has little if any effect on breathing. Exercise of this intensity will increase your heart rate to 40–55% of its maximum. In a 50-year-old this would be between 68 and 94 beats per minute (40–55% of 170). Although exercise of this intensity will not significantly improve your cardiovascular fitness or result in significant weight reduction, it will, if done frequently and for long enough, favourably alter the risks of developing cardiovascular disease, high blood pressure and diabetes. This is sometimes referred to as 'metabolic fitness' (as opposed to cardiovascular fitness).

MODERATE-INTENSITY EXERCISE (Level 2)

Exercise of this intensity results in some shortness of breath so that continuous conversation is just possible. This level of exercise will increase your heart rate to 55–70% of your maximum heart rate. In our example of a 50-year-old this would be 94–119 beats per minute (55–70% of 170). This sort of exercise level can be achieved even by brisk walking and is suitable for people with coronary artery disease. In addition to achieving metabolic fitness, it will result in weight reduction and increased cardiovascular fitness.

HIGH-INTENSITY EXERCISE (Level 3)

With this level of exercise intensity a normal continuous conversation is not possible (and if you were considering whistling the theme of *Bridge Over the River Kwai* you'd find it difficult). This level of exercise will increase your heart rate to 70–90% or more of its maximum. In our example of the 50-year-old, this would be 119–153 beats per minute (70–90% of 170). With regular training this is achievable. At this level you'll enhance fat burning and achieve weight reduction and a high level of cardiovascular fitness. Because higher-intensity exercise is associated with a greater cardiovascular risk, it's advisable to work up to these levels in a gradual way.

Heart rate targets (percentage of maximum heart rate)					
Age	50%	60%	75%	85%	90%
40	90	108	135	153	162
45	87	105	131	149	158
50	85	102	128	145	153
55	83	99	124	140	149
60	80	96	120	136	144
65	78	93	116	132	140
70	75	90	113	128	135
75	73	87	109	122	131
80	70	84	105	119	126
85	68	81	101	115	122

HOW TO DETERMINE YOUR STARTING LEVEL FOR CARDIOVASCULAR TRAINING

Remember the resistance training levels in Chapter 13? Well, the same principles apply to cardiovascular training. However, your resistance training level and cardiovascular training level may be quite different, depending on such factors as age, body weight, and current fitness level. For example, you may be at cardiovascular training Level 3 but be at resistance training Level 1. Of course, the ultimate is to be at Level 3 in both. This requires some effort but is achievable. All it requires is commitment. The level at which you begin is not important. Getting started is. Remember you are not in a competition against anyone else. You're training for your life, not someone else's.

Identifying the level for you
PRE-LEVEL 1 (low intensity)
This is recommended:

(1) For the 60–90-year-old age group, particularly those of you who've never previously done any regular exercise (resistance or cardiovascular), and for those who may have last exercised some time ago.

(2) For those with severe arthritis (Functional Class 3 and some in Functional Class 2—see Chapter 7).

LEVEL 1 (low intensity)
This is recommended:

(1) For those under 60 years who may never have done any regular exercise (resistance or cardiovascular), and for those who may have last exercised some time ago.

(2) For those with mild to moderate arthritis.

LEVEL 2 (moderate intensity)
This is recommended:

(1) For those who've been doing some form of regular exercise, such as a sporting activity with a significant cardiovascular component (e.g. squash, jogging, fast cycling, swimming, rowing) or resistance training. This may include some people with mild arthritis who have been regular exercisers.

LEVEL 3 (high intensity)
This is recommended:

(1) For those who have already achieved a high level of fitness through regular cardiovascular training or a sporting activity with a significant cardiovascular component. If you have been training regularly but are uncertain of just how fit you are, it is recommended that you make a start at Level 2 even if for only 6 weeks, before moving on to Level 3. The details of the various cardiovascular training levels are described in Chapter 16.

Cardiovascular fitness works roughly like this: the more time you spend training at a particular level the sooner that will become your fitness level.

HOW TO GET THERE

There are a number of ways to improve your cardiovascular fitness level. The emphasis in this program is on low-impact aerobic training, which includes such activities as walking and cycling, and using an exercise bike, treadmill, stepper, versaclimber, rower or cross-trainer. High-impact endurance training, such as running and aerobics that involve jumping, are associated with a higher risk of injury, not only in beginners but also in experienced exercisers. This form of training is not recommended for older adults or for people with arthritis.

Running

Some of you may ask, 'What about running?'. As I mentioned in Chapter 1, I'm an ex-long-distance runner. I absolutely loved the sport. There was a time in my life when I couldn't have imagined life without running. Then my knees let me down. If I wanted to keep exercising I had to find an alternative, and I did. This has not turned me against running but it's important to understand that older knee joints (in particular) are much less tolerant of the stresses of running than are younger knee joints, for reasons already discussed. In fact there are published scientific studies that suggest that osteoarthritis in the knees may occur at a relatively early age in adult life in those who've played certain sports, including soccer, rugby, racquet sports and track and field sports. If you are not overweight and have straight legs (as opposed to being bandy-legged or knock-kneed), then you're less likely to develop knee joint problems. If you're aged 40 or older and haven't been a regular runner, then my personal view is that there are safer ways of cardiovascular training than taking up running later in life. These days there are some great cardiovascular machines available in most gyms and I hope you'll keep an open mind on expanding your cardiovascular training horizons.

Another thing—if you are a woman, distance running won't prevent osteoporosis.

In the over-40 age group the risk of joint problems and injury in runners is high, particularly if you are heavy-framed. If you have an unshakable desire to continue running then you might consider treadmill running, which is much kinder on the joints.

Walking

Some people have suggested that walking is an over-rated exercise. This may be because for some time now people have been given unreal expectations of the benefits of walking. One of these expectations was that walking could prevent osteoporosis. However a study that compared bone density in women on a high-intensity training program with women who walked for exercise found that the walking group actually *lost* bone density. Some people interpreted these data as meaning that walking simply wasn't any good for anything. This is not so. There's one group for whom walking is definitely not over-rated and that is those with coronary artery disease. Guidelines in Australia and in the United States for physical activity in people with coronary artery disease recommend an accumulation of at least 30 minutes of moderate-intensity physical activity on most and preferably all days of the week.

Moderate-intensity activity is covered by brisk, not slow, walking and/or by resistance training. A recent study of more than 7000 men with an average age of 66 years who walked and exercised regularly showed a significant reduction in factors known to increase the risk of coronary heart disease. This included a lowering of blood pressure, a reduction in the likelihood of blood clots forming, and an increase in the body's sensitivity to insulin. This study also found that it was unnecessary to exercise for long periods—accumulating a number of shorter sessions in a day was just as protective as one longer session.

Exercise scientists point out that, while any activity is better than none, much exercise time is wasted if it's not sufficiently intense. As we increase the intensity of exercise, the body gradually burns more carbohydrate than fat. This has led some to suggest that the reverse holds true—namely that low intensity exercise is best for fat burning. This is undoubtedly the reason why at any time of the day or night one can see overweight people walking gently along the road. If you were say a visitor from Mars you might be forgiven for thinking that walking caused earthlings to become obese. However, low-intensity exercise is not useless. It will deliver substantial health benefits but we now know that it's necessary to increase the intensity of exercising in order to enhance the body's ability to burn fat. This will not happen with gentle walking. It will happen with moderate to high-intensity exercise. It will happen as you increase your lean body mass (your muscle).

Studies indicate that for a 90 kilogram male to lose any weight would require almost five hours of walking a week and for a 70 kilogram woman about six hours a week. For most people this would constitute a significant time commitment. Other data indicate that, even with the addition of weights carried at shoulder level, there's only a very marginal effect on the demands of the exercise.

For some time it was considered that gentle walking was the only safe exercise for people with coronary artery disease. However we now know that brisk walking and resistance training of varied intensity are safe for this group.

Walking will:
■ reduce the risk of developing coronary heart disease
■ lower blood pressure
■ reduce the risk of diabetes.

Walking will not:
■ build muscle (except in your legs, and in your arms if you 'powerwalk')
■ prevent osteoporosis
■ result in significant weight loss.

The advantage of cardiovascular machines is that at the press of a button or the turning of a dial you can alter their resistance. This means that you are able to increase the intensity of the exercise and thus maximise the benefits from your exercise time. You can even change the resistance in the course of your exercise, or you can maintain the same resistance and simply increase the speed at which you are working—all very convenient. Begin all of your cardiovascular machine training sessions with a 2 to 3 minute warm-up before gradually increasing the tempo of your exercise for whatever period of time you've decided beforehand, and then end your session with a 2 to 3 minute cool-down.

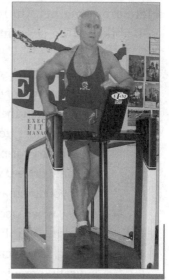

TREADMILL

This is a machine with a moving track on which you can walk or run. The speed of the track can be varied to suit your level of fitness and your exercise goals. The advantage over road running or walking is that there's much less jarring to the joints of the legs. Treadmills have side-support bars in case you lose your balance, and most have a visual display screen indicating the training intensity level, distance covered and elapsed time.

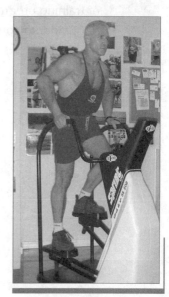

STEPPER

This is a machine with rubber or plastic foot plates which move as you 'step'. It has support bars for safety and a visual display screen, indicating the training intensity level, number of steps taken per minute, distance covered and time elapsed.

EXERCISE BIKE

Most people have ridden a pedal bike at some stage in life.
Dead-easy, isn't it? An exercise bike is even easier because you
don't need to worry about losing your balance or avoiding traffic.
This leaves time to concentrate on proper riding technique.
Here are some helpful hints to enable you to get the most out of
your bike riding session:

- *First*, adjust the seat to the correct height by making sure that
  your knee is only slightly bent at the bottom of your pedal stroke.
- *Next*, tighten the pedal straps over your shoes. This will help to
  stop your feet from coming off the pedals but more importantly
  is necessary for proper pedalling technique, which requires that you
  not only drive down with your legs but that you also lift your legs
  (as if you are marking time with a high knee lift).
- *Finally*, when pedalling concentrate on keeping your face muscles,
  jaw, arms and shoulders relaxed, and try to control your breathing
  as long as you can. Exercise bikes have a visual display screen
  indicating training intensity level, distance covered and time
  elapsed and also offer a choice
  of training program
  (e.g. random course or
  hill climb).

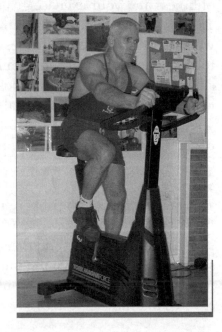

CROSS-TRAINER

This is a machine which simulates cross-country skiing and involves simultaneously moving the legs and arms. As with other cardiovascular machines, it has a visual display screen indicating the training intensity level, distance covered and time elapsed.

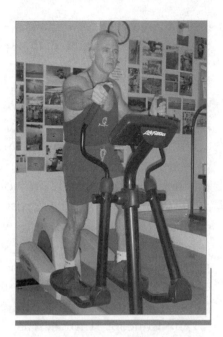

VERSA-CLIMBER

This is one of the great cardiovascular machines. It's really a stepper with pedals and overhead horizontal handles. The pedals and handles work at the same time so that as you press down on the pedal the handle on the same side is pulled downwards. If you place additional downward force on the handle while simultaneously depressing the pedal, you can increase the speed at which you climb. A visual display indicates elapsed time, number of metres or feet climbed per minute, and total distance climbed.

This is a great machine for increasing cardiovascular fitness and improving leg and arm strength. In the beginning you may have difficulty in climbing faster than 33 metres a minute (100 feet a minute), but as you get fitter and stronger your speed will increase and eventually you may be able to climb

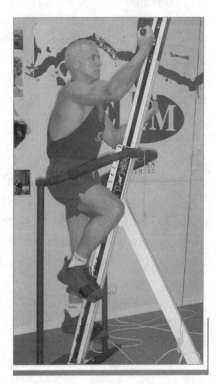

faster than 66 metres a minute (about 200 feet a minute). Only the very fittest are able to maintain this speed for more than 3 to 4 minutes.

ROWER

This is my favourite piece of cardiovascular equipment. The Concept II rower is simple, 'idiot proof' and never breaks down. Because it accurately simulates rowing in the water it's used worldwide by professional and recreational rowers and scullers of all standards. Furthermore, because it provides a total body workout, it's used by athletes in all sports for 'cross-training'. It has a simple-to-operate computer that is set before you start your row. A small screen provides information on total distance rowed, elapsed time, strokes per minute and real-time speed per 500 metres. These readings are continuously displayed on the screen (you don't have to stop rowing to press a button to get the information).

The Concept II rower has been described as the complete body workout because at the same time as improving your cardiovascular fitness, you're getting resistance training to your arms and legs. For further information check the Concept II website at www.concept2.com.

HOW TO ROW

As with resistance training, technique and breathing are all-important for getting the most benefit out of the exercise. With proper technique you will: (1) row faster, (2) row further, (3) not waste energy, and (4) not run the risk of injury.

There are two phases to the rowing stroke, the *drive* and the *recovery*, which are best described as a number of steps, though the movements are blended together to make the stroke smooth and continuous. There should be no stopping at any point in the stroke.

Step 1.

Reach forward with knees bent, arms extended and body leaning forward towards the fly wheel. *Do not bend your back*. The drive is begun with the legs and the back doing all the work. Before beginning the drive your arms should be straight and your shoulders relaxed, and you shouldn't be gripping the handle tightly.

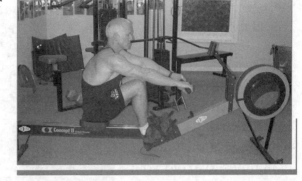

Step 2.
Drive back in a smooth motion by accelerating through the drive—don't jerk the handle towards you. Push off your toes and straighten your legs. Halfway through the drive, your arms should still be straight (they only start to bend after they have passed above your knees). Breathe in during this phase of the rowing stroke.

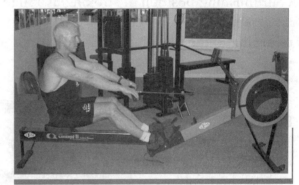

Step 3.
At the finish of the drive breathe out and pull the handle into the upper abdomen (not the chest). At this point your legs are straight and your body is leaning back but only slightly.

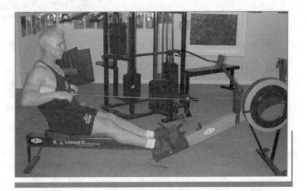

Step 4.
This is the recovery
phase and is begun by
extending the arms and
allowing the body to
move forward at the
hips. The handle should
be in front of the knees
at all times to avoid your
bent knees obstructing
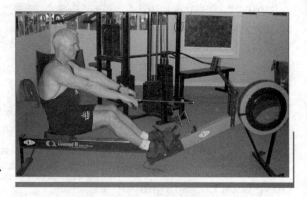
the smooth passage of the handle to its starting position. During the
recovery phase, breathe in and then breathe out just as you reach
your finishing position. If stroking at a high rate you may find it
necessary on the recovery phase to breathe in and out twice before
returning to the finishing position.

Step 5.
Your finishing position is
identical to your starting
position and you're
ready for your next
stroke.
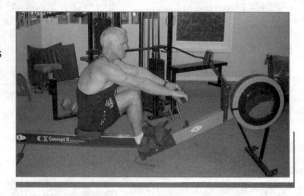

The training variations on the rower are infinite. For example
you can row continuously and steadily for a prolonged period of
time or you can do interval training by varying your speed for a
particular distance or time interval. Further information on training
schedules can be obtained from www.concept2.com.

Water-based exercise

Swimming and water aerobics are especially suitable for people with arthritis, particularly where there is a very limited range of joint movement. Exercises in water minimise weight bearing and allow for a greater range of joint movement while providing some resistance. However there is only so much that can be achieved with water-based exercises alone. A goal should be to try to graduate to resistance exercises out of the water. Of course not everyone has access to a swimming pool and cost may be an issue.

Circuit weight training

This involves training with moderate weights almost continuously using 10–20 reps per exercise, with no more than 15–30 seconds' rest between the exercises. Studies have shown that this results in only a modest improvement in cardiovascular fitness unless combined with cardiovascular exercise (e.g. treadmill, exercise bike, rower, stepper, cross-trainer, versa-climber). Thus, circuit weight training alone is not recommended as the only activity for developing cardiovascular fitness.

HOW TO STAY THERE

To maintain the training effect you will need to continue to train on a regular basis. However, you need not become neurotic about missing an occasional training session, providing it's only occasional and providing that when you do train you keep up your usual intensity. In maintaining cardiovascular fitness, training *intensity* is more important than training frequency or duration. Having said this, frequency and duration are of course important. A complete break of two weeks, for example, will result in a reduction in cardiovascular fitness, and a break of 10 weeks or longer will result in a return to near pre-training levels of fitness.

Chapter 16

Cardiovascular
training
programs

| '*It is the effort you make
to improve yourself that
is measured.*'

MIYAMOTO MUSASHI,
THE BOOK OF FIVE RINGS

TRAINING PROGRAM FOR PRE-LEVEL 1 (low intensity)

- Try to have a minimum of four to five training sessions per week.
- For the first three weeks, exercise at 40–50% of your maximum heart rate (MHR) for 20 minutes. If necessary this can be broken up into two 10-minute sessions.
- For the next three weeks or longer, exercise at 40–50% of your MHR for 30 minutes. If necessary this can be broken up into three 10-minute sessions.
- When you feel ready, move on to Level 1.

Research suggests that the benefits of exercise are related to total quantity of activity, even if activity is undertaken in relatively short bursts. Remember what we discussed earlier? Accumulating a number of shorter sessions can be as beneficial as fewer longer sessions at Pre-Level 1. If you happen to fall into the 'low-fit' category, this six weeks low-intensity starting phase will allow for adaptation with minimal risk of injury. Even if towards the end of the six weeks everything seems too easy, I advise you to complete this phase of your training before progressing to the next level. Generally after that you can safely increase your exercise intensity and, if you wish, decrease your exercise time.

TRAINING PROGRAM FOR LEVEL 1 (low intensity)

- Try to have a minimum of three training sessions per week.
- For the first three weeks, exercise at 50% of your MHR for 40 minutes. If necessary this can be broken up into two to four sessions in a day.
- For the next three weeks or longer, exercise at 55% of your MHR for up to 60 minutes. If necessary this can be broken up into three 20-minute sessions in a day.
- When you feel ready, move on to Level 2.

TRAINING PROGRAM FOR LEVEL 2 (moderate intensity)

- Try to have a minimum of 2 training sessions per week.
- For the first three weeks, exercise continuously at 60% of your MHR for at least 20 minutes.
- For the next three weeks or longer, exercise continuously at 65–70% of your MHR for at least 20 minutes.
- When you feel ready, move on to Level 3.

TRAINING PROGRAM FOR LEVEL 3 (high intensity)

- Try to have a minimum of 2 training sessions per week.
- For the first three weeks or longer, exercise continuously at 80% of your MHR for at least 20 minutes.
- When you feel ready, try to increase your exercise intensity above 80% of your MHR for varying periods of time in a training session lasting 30 minutes or longer
- At Level 3, you may wish to introduce interval training sessions. Try this interval training program on the rower, exercise bike, treadmill, stepper or versa-climber:

    (example 50-year-old athlete)

    50% of MHR x 2 min (85 beats per minute)

    80% of MHR x 1 min (136 beats per minute)

    85% of MHR x 1 min (145 beats per minute)

    90% of MHR x 1 min (153 beats per minute)

    50% of MHR x 1 min

    80% of MHR x 1 min

85% of MHR x 1 min
90% of MHR x 1 min
50% of MHR x 30 sec
80% of MHR x 1 min
85% of MHR x 1 min
90% of MHR x 1 min
50% of MHR x 30 sec
80% of MHR x 1 min
85% of MHR x 1 min
90% of MHR x 1 min

Remember to cool down with 2–3 minutes of easy activity on whatever machine you're using.

HOW LONG PER SESSION?

You will have noticed that the lower the training intensity level the longer the recommended training session. Pre-Level 1 exercisers may initially find they have to break up cardiovascular training periods, but these should last a minimum of 10 minutes. A goal should be to try to achieve at least 20 minutes continuously and to accumulate between 40 and 60 minutes in a day. At moderate to high intensity levels a minimum of 20 minutes is recommended. This is because studies have shown that to obtain an optimal cardiovascular benefit requires at least 20 minutes of cardiovascular exercise.

HOW OFTEN PER WEEK?

The American College of Sports Medicine suggests that to achieve a satisfactory and reliable training effect requires two to three cardiovascular training sessions per week. Exercise at lower intensity levels needs to be undertaken more frequently than exercise of moderate or high intensity. Level 2 and Level 3 exercisers should aim for at least two cardiovascular training sessions and two resistance training sessions per week. Many of the physical, psychological and social benefits of exercise require this level of activity.

THE PRE-LEVEL 1 AND LEVEL 1 DILEMMA

The cardiovascular program for Pre-Level 1 recommends four to five training sessions per week, lasting for up to 30 minutes per session, and for Level 1 three training sessions per week lasting up to 60 minutes per session. These programs are in line with the cardiovascular training recommendations of the American College of Sports Medicine but they do impose a significant time commitment. The dilemma is finding the time to accommodate these programs and the resistance training program into a a one-week training cycle. It can be done if you're prepared to exercise six or seven days a week, but even for low-intensity exercisers the time commitment is likely to become a drag. One solution is to have a 10-day training cycle but this, it must be said, is less convenient and can get confusing.

My advice for Pre-Level 1 exercisers is to sacrifice resistance training for cardiovascular training for your first six weeks and concentrate only on the cardiovascular training. By then you'll probably be able to move to Level 1, where the cardiovascular commitment drops to three sessions and you could accommodate one or two resistance training sessions per week. If at six weeks you don't feel ready to move from Pre-Level 1 to Level 1, drop back to three or four cardiovascular sessions and make a start on the resistance training program. Of course, once you reach Level 2 or Level 3 the cardiovascular training requirements fall to two sessions anyway and there is then no difficulty in accommodating at least two resistance training sessions per week.

Chapter 17

Back pain
and
back exercises

> *'There is no convincing, let alone indisputable evidence that low back pain is more prevalent in the workplace broadly defined, in any particular industry or in any particular type of work. The inescapable conclusion is that backache is a nearly universal predicament.'*

NORTIN HADLER

If you're over the age of 40 and have never had an episode of low back pain, then you are abnormal! You're also very lucky, because population studies indicate that back pain is a predicament shared by 80% of people at some stage in life—irrespective of occupation or sporting activities. As a matter of fact, between one-quarter and one-third of adults are likely to be actually experiencing low back pain at the time they are surveyed!

Remember in Chapter 2 we discussed how by age 50 more than 85% of people have X-ray evidence of degenerative changes in their lower back (lumbar) region. That's pretty close to the 80% figure of people who experience backache at some stage in life. So the logical conclusion is that the cause of low back pain in that 80% is the degenerative changes we know are to be found in 85% of people.

Some things however seem to defy logic. You see, when we compare X-rays of people who have low back pain with X-rays of those without back pain, and match them for age, there is no difference. That's right, the X-ray appearance of your spine will not predict whether you are a candidate for low back pain. In fact, some people who are troubled by chronic low back pain have completely normal X-rays for their age! It follows therefore that there must be another factor responsible, and of course there is. Actually there may be a number of factors but we've identified the most important and the most common one—and it just happens to be a factor that we can do something about.

I'm talking about a *corset*—except that you won't have to go out and buy one. You already have it. If you're troubled by recurring low back pain, chances are your corset is not being used properly and/or it's gone out of shape. Exactly what am I talking about? I am talking about the body's natural 'corset', which is a complex, interlacing web of abdominal and back muscle fibres, ligaments and fascia (connecting tissue).

THE TRANSVERSUS ABDOMINIS

Don't you love it when you go to your doctor complaining of low back pain and you're told to exercise your tummy muscles? Well, that's right—but it ain't that simple! You see, the only abdominal muscle that is attached to the lumbar fascia (connecting tissue in the lower back) is a deep abdominal muscle—the transversus abdominis (we will refer to this as the 'TA'). Because the TA attaches to the lumbar fascia (which in turn attaches to the lumbar muscles), when the TA tightens the 'corset' tightens. The thing is you can't see the TA—it's not one of the abs muscles which contribute to the '6 pack' nor even to the '8 pack'. These are the superficial abdominal muscles (rectus abdominis and internal and external obliques). It's possible to have great, rippling abs and still have back pain because of a weak TA.

You won't strengthen your TA with sit-ups, which is why I don't recommend them. You *will* strengthen your TA with crunches, but only if while doing them you draw your belly button up and backwards towards your spine. If you do crunches this way, you will work both your TA and your superficial abdominal muscles. You will get your 6 pack as well as a strong 'corset'.

Acquiring control of your TA can be difficult. If you have chronic low back pain you may need to consult a physiotherapist for special instruction on how to bring your TA into action. It can take a few sessions.

EXERCISES FOR BACK PAIN

If you have low back pain, or a history of recurrent episodes of low back pain, then in addition to the abs and back exercises described in Chapter 12 you should also do these exercises:

1. TA PRIMER

Lie on the floor with your knees bent. Place your hands above your hips, thumbs facing backwards and fingers slightly downwards and towards your belly button. Now breathe in while pushing your 'stomach' out (beer-belly style) and then while breathing out pull your belly button up and backwards towards your spine. As you do this you'll feel your lower abs muscles push into your fingers. Hold this position to a count of 10. As you 'gain control' of your TA you'll be able to hold this position for longer periods.

Having a pillow under your head, or slightly lifting your shoulders off the floor, can make this exercise easier to master.

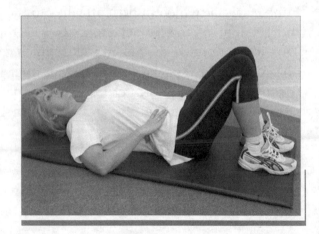

2. PARTIAL SIT-UP

Lie on the floor with your knees bent and your hands resting on your thighs. Flatten out your back by tilting your pubic bone towards your chin and pull your belly button up and backwards towards your

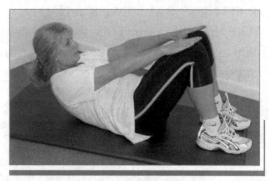

spine. Remember the imaginary 20c piece (from Chapter 12)? Then sit up until your hands just slide over your knees. Stop. Hold this for 10 seconds and then relax. Repeat. In time, you should be able to maintain the hold for up to 30 seconds and increase the number of repetitions.

3. FITNESS BALL BACK ROLL

Sit upright on the ball with your knees bent at 100–120°. Roll the ball backwards until the ball is under your shoulders, then pause in this position for 10 seconds without allowing your hips to sag. Return to your starting position.

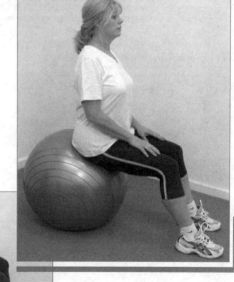

4. FITNESS BALL BACK PADDLE

With the ball under your shoulders simultaneously raise your right arm and your left leg. Hold for 5 seconds and repeat with the opposite arm and leg.

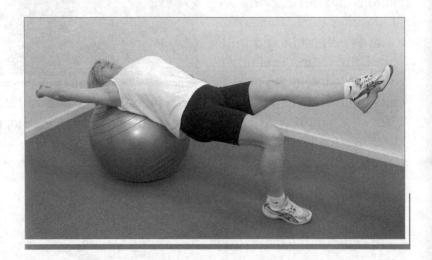

Chapter **18** Kicking
goals

> '*It is said that one should not hesitate to correct himself when he has made a mistake. If he corrects himself without the least bit of delay his mistakes will quickly disappear.'*
>
> YAMAMOTO TSUNOMOTO,
> *THE BOOK OF THE SAMURAI* (HAGAKURE)

THE IMPORTANCE OF GOALS

It is important at the outset to have a goal you've determined for yourself. Do not be influenced by other people's goals and do not let other people set goals for you. You will quickly tire of trying to meet someone else's expectations.

Sit down quietly and decide just what it is you'd like to get out of your training and eating program. Remember, your goal isn't a fantasy—it is something you can turn into a reality. Use the '90% rule' to determine whether your goal is realistic or not. This rule considers the goal to be realistic if you are at least 90% sure you can achieve it. Your goal is yours alone. It is a personal thing that you may or may not wish to share with someone. It is often helpful to write down your goals and to visualise them.

Do not set multiple goals initially. New habits, even healthy ones like exercise and dietary modification, take time to develop. It is best to focus on one or two short-term goals—something you can achieve within eight to 12 weeks. These don't have to be earth-shatteringly ambitious. For example, a reasonable goal might be to attend a minimum of two sessions a week for eight weeks and then three sessions a week after that. Another goal might be to move from Level 1 to Level 2 within a particular time frame. You may have a slightly longer-term goal, for example to lose weight. You may want to lose weight and build a better body. Some people may want to actually gain weight by increasing their lean body mass (muscle). It may be that you have heart disease or a family history of heart disease and wish to reduce risk factors. You may want to reduce the risk of osteoporosis, diabetes or cancer. You may simply want to reduce your stress levels. If you have arthritis, your goal may be to improve your range of joint movement and to stabilise your joints by building the muscle around the joints. If you are an older adult, your goal may be to remain independent for as long as possible. The point is, *your goal is yours*. The nature of your goal is less important than your formulating it and committing to it. And, once you've achieved your goals, *write down your achievements*.

COPING WITH SET-BACKS
In older adults and in people with arthritis who are exercising regularly, set-backs are almost inevitable. In fact, set-backs are the rule rather than the exception. These can take many forms.

INJURY FAILURE
We discussed previously how as we get older our 'anchoring tissues' (ligaments and tendons) are prone to injury. To reduce the likelihood of injury to these tissues, remember our earlier principles: choose the right weight, begin your program gradually, and lift and lower weights with good form. If you do happen to get injured acutely, apply ice and, if necessary, see a doctor. You may still be able to exercise the injured muscle by using a lighter weight or by doing a different exercise for that muscle group. If it is necessary to rest the injured part, then you may still be able to exercise other muscle groups.

Remember, injuries are common—don't lose heart.

SESSION FAILURE

Try to keep to your training days. Sometimes however it's impossible to get there for one reason or another. Sometimes we experience a lapse of resolve—it happens. But a temporary lapse from activity does not mean you're a failure. Lapses are normal. Don't be discouraged. Don't feel guilty. Don't engage in all-or-none thinking—'I've missed two sessions this week—that's it—I'm finished'. Have you ever ridden a horse? Almost everyone who's ridden a horse has fallen off—not once but several times. If they said, 'That's it—I'm done—I'll never ride again', I imagine there would be very few people riding horses today. The idea is to get back on as soon as possible, just as if you miss a training session try to resume your training as soon as possible. You'll feel better about yourself and regain your confidence.

DIET FAILURE

OK—so you're human. We all enjoy food but not everything we enjoy is good for us. You're allowed a weekly lapse—but try to keep it to only one day of the week. And eat what you like. This is your 'safety valve' day and it needn't be a day on which you're working out. You haven't failed, you've just been normal—join the club.

GOAL FAILURE

To have achieved your goal may have required sustained, high-intensity activity or at least a level of activity you've found very difficult to sustain. You feel the doubts creeping in. Don't throw the whole thing away because you feel you haven't or won't achieve your hoped-for goal. Despite the '90% rule' your initial goal may have just been too ambitious—it happens. All you did was miscalculate. Think of this as losing a skirmish—you haven't lost the war. It's no reason to run up the white flag. Fall back, regroup and try a different strategy.

ADDRESSING GOAL FAILURE

There are a number of measures you can employ to get yourself back on track:

1. Try lowering your lifting weights for one or two weeks. Then, keeping your weights the same, increase your reps. At the end of the day you won't have lost much, if anything.

2. If you've seriously miscalculated your goal (this is usually unlikely with the '90% rule'), you may have to drop back a training level, for example from Level 1 to Pre-Level 1 or from Level 2 to Level 1. Remember, low (as opposed to moderate or high) intensity activity will still provide you with substantial health benefits.

3. Use the 'mini-goal' strategy to deal with a set-back. This may be as simple as getting through your weekly sessions, even if you've had to lower the intensity of your sessions.

RIGHT THINKING

I mentioned at the beginning of this book that I'd been a marathoner and martial artist—very different pursuits but linked by a common thread. Both require a degree of commitment and resolve. After that, the hardest part of marathon running is getting out of bed to make the morning run. Once you're out on the road it becomes easier. In martial arts it's getting to the dojo (the training place), and this is hard mainly because in most western countries training is held in the evening—after you've had a long, hard day. Like running, once you get there and get going it just happens.

If you have the ability and discipline to get out of bed every morning to go to work or to meet other commitments, then you have the necessary prerequisites of commitment and resolve to train for a long and healthy life. It's as simple as that.

Sometimes it helps to have a particular mental approach. Think of yourself as a warrior. Training is integral to your existence. It's what you do—just like going to work or brushing your teeth. The time required to do it needs to be factored into your life. And, when you've had a big night (or a late one) or a lousy day at work or you're 'feeling weak' or even miserable—turn up. Those training sessions when you feel below peak are often the most satisfying—the thing is you have to do them to find this out.

HOW DO I KNOW IF I'M GETTING ANYWHERE?

Chances are the people you know will notice something different about you and will tell you that you're 'looking well' or 'fitter'. From your own point of view it's important that you measure your progress from your starting point. If you haven't exercised for some time it would be unreasonable to expect to pick up from the point where you left off, particularly if you were previously exercising regularly. When resuming exercise after years of doing very little, the first thing you'll notice is that you become breathless more quickly and that you're not quite as strong as you were previously. Relax, this is entirely normal. Remember that, whatever your age, there is plenty of room for substantial gains in strength and fitness. Don't get disheartened because you feel that your first few training sessions are difficult. They will be. Stick with your program and then assess the situation after eight weeks. You won't look back.

SELF-REWARDS

Reinforce your goals by self-rewards. Make these dependent on meeting a particular training goal. The rewards might include anything from going out to a favourite restaurant, going away for the weekend or buying yourself a new CD.

It's also important to review your goals. They shouldn't be seen as something static. For example, once you've achieved your goals you may wish to commit to a new set of goals. This is entirely appropriate. These new goals may include simply continuing what you've already been doing, or you may wish to increase your weights and build more strength or increase your muscle mass. You may even wish to reduce or modify goals that were overly ambitious.

THE DECISION

Well, that's my story. Now I guess it's up to you to decide whether you want to try to put into practice what you've read. I sincerely hope that many of you will take the plunge or, at the very least, dip your toe into the shallow end. To all who decide to 'have a go', I wish you a long, healthy and happy life.

Further
resources

'Live Stronger—Live Longer'
Visit the website on live-stronger-live-longer.com
T-Shirt—A$30.00
Singlet/vest A$27.50
(includes postage in Australia; for orders outside of Australia
add A$7.50)

Buying equipment
Cost of weights +/- A$1.00 per pound or A$2.50 per kilogram
Cost of bench A$120.00
Cost of Concept II Rower A$2,288.00
Cost of Therabands (resistance bands) +/- A$8.00 per metre
Cost of Polar heart rate monitor A$99.00–A$500.00 (depending on how
sophisticated you want to be)

Arthritis Foundation of Australia
All state and territory foundations listed below are affiliated with the
Arthritis Foundation of Australia. They offer a wide range of services and
information to their members and welcome new members to their branches
and self-help groups throughout Australia. The National Arthritis
Information Line is 1800 011 041 and there's a full list of branches and
groups at www.arthritisfoundation.com.au.

Arthritis Foundation of New South Wales: 13 Harold Street
North Parramatta NSW 2151
Locked Bag 16, PO
North Parramatta NSW 2151
Tel: (02) 9683 1622

Arthritis Foundation of Victoria:	263-265 Kooyong Road
	Elsternwick VIC 3185
	PO BOX 130
	Caulfield South VIC 3162
	Tel: (03) 9530 0255
Arthritis Foundation of Queensland:	PO BOX 807
	Spring Hill QLD 4004
	Tel: (07) 3831 4255
Arthritis Foundation of South Australia:	Unit 1, 202-208 Glen Osmond Rd
	Fullarton SA 5063
	Tel: (08) 8379 5771
Arthritis Foundation of Western Australia:	17 Lemnos Street
	Shenton Park WA 6008
	PO BOX 34
	Wembley WA 6014
	Tel: (08) 9388 2199
Arthritis Foundation of Tasmania:	Box 30, McDougall Blvd
	Ellerslie Road
	Battery Point TAS 7004
	Tel: (03) 6234 6489
Arthritis Foundation of ACT:	Health Promotions Centre
	Childers Street
	Canberra City ACT 2600
	GPO BOX 1642
	Canberra ACT 2601
	Tel: (02) 6257 4842
Arthritis Foundation of Northern Territory:	Nightcliff Community Centre
	18 Bauhinia Street
	Nightcliff NT 0810
	Tel: (08) 8948 5232

Fitness Australia

Fitness Australia is the peak body in Australia for accreditation of fitness instructors. Each state, and the ACT, has its own branch. The gyms listed below are only those that are affiliated with these state branches. For information on other gyms consult the *Yellow Pages* or call the state or territory branch of Fitness Australia. If you are interested in a particular gym it's worth calling to see if it has specific programs for older exercisers. The state/territory contacts are as follows:

Fitness ACT	Stephen Butler	(02) 6248 5934
Fitness NSW	Ian Grainger	(02) 9460 6200
Fitness QLD	Gordon McDonald	(07) 3876 6522
Fitness SA	Kathy Ayliffe	(08) 8272 8399
Fitness TAS	Terry Curtain	(03) 6224 8324
Fitness WA	Ros Howell	(08) 9383 7734
Fitness VIC	Phillip Staindl	(03) 9428 7733

In Victoria, Karen Byrush is the co-ordinator of a project run by Council on the Aging. The project is called 'Living Longer Living Stronger' and specifically addresses the needs of older exercisers. The contact number is (03) 9654 4443.

Gyms affiliated with Fitness Australia in each state
For phone numbers of other gyms consult the **Yellow Pages** *or call the branch of Fitness Australia in your state or territory.*

ACT

NAME	SUBURB	PHONE
ACT Fitness Connection	Mitchell	(02) 6258 1689
Active Leisure Centre	Wanniassa	(02) 6207 2777
Advantage Fitness Consultancy	Queanbeyan	(02) 6297 4027
Advantage Personal Trainers	Queanbeyan	0402 451 049
AIS Health & Fitness Centre	Belconnen	(02) 6214 1652
ANU Sports Union	Canberra City	(02) 6249 4808
Belconnen Fitness Centre	Belconnen	(02) 6253 1166
Bodyworks Fitness	Belconnen	(02) 6251 4338
	Kaleen	(02) 6241 3622
	Mawson	(02) 6290 1902

City YMCA	Canberra City	(02) 6249 8733
Deakin Health Spa	Deakin	(02) 6285 2514
Ele's Refit: Rehabilitation	Woden	0413 338 420
Fernwood Belconnen	Belconnen	(02) 6251 5299
Fernwood Fitness Centre	Braddon	(02) 6247 7666
Fit and Healthy	Jamison	(02) 6251 5975
Fit Happens Personal Training	Forrest	0411 850 560
Fitness First	All suburbs	0414 538 348
Fitness One	Canberra City	(02) 6284 3330
Flames Fitness	North Lyneham	(02) 6257 1483
Fun & Fitness Personal Trainers	All suburbs	(02) 6231 5888
Gold Creek Country Club	Harcourt Hill	(02) 6241 9888
Inshape Health Club	Canberra City	(02) 6248 6799
Inshape Health Club	Tuggeranong	(02) 6293 3122
Jazzercise – Northside	O'Connor	(02) 6248 9136
Jazzercise – Tuggeranong	Kambah	(02) 6231 2044
JT's Fitness Centre	Goulburn (NSW)	(02) 4821 5024
Nick A'Hern Fitness	Manukah	(02) 6260 8500
Northside Fitness Centre	Dickson	(02) 6247 7893
Oasis Leisure Centre	Deakin	(02) 6281 1535
Odd Bods Fitness Centre	Queanbeyan	(02) 6297 7788
Oulgeah Centre	Deakin	(02) 6281 1819
Peak Performance Personal Training	Duffy	0418 881 615
Planet Action	Dickson	(02) 6247 8930
Pro Fitness	Scullen	(02) 6254 8615
Queanbeyan Leagues Club Gymnasium	Queanbeyan	(02) 6297 2511
Shape and Squash Fitness Centre	Goulburn (NSW)	(02) 4821 5024
Southern Cross Health & Fitness Centre	Woden	(02) 6283 7340
Sportsfolio	Queanbeyan	(02) 6299 7750
The Canberra Club	Canberra City	(02) 6248 9000
The Club House	Yarralumla	(02) 6269 8540
The Fitness Edge	Mawson	(02) 6286 9844

Tuggeranong Community Centre	Tuggeranong	(02) 6293 2942
UCU Recreation Centre	Bruce	(02) 6201 2542
Underground Gym Centre	Weston	(02) 6287 3707
Vikings Health & Fitness Centre	Erindale	(02) 6231 6597
Vital Action	Belconnen	(02) 6251 5161
Weston Creek Community Centre	Weston	(02) 6288 1144
Yass Community Centre	Yass (NSW)	(02) 6226 3833
YMCA Jamison	Macquarie	(02) 6251 1683

NEW SOUTH WALES

NAME	SUBURB	PHONE
Ace Fitness	Lavington	(02) 6040 2377
Active Fitness	North Ryde	(02) 9878 5595
Adfit	Menai	(02) 9543 1500
Ausbodz Fitness Centre	Parramatta	(02) 9687 1616
Balmain Fitness	Rozelle	(02) 9818 3555
Bayswater Fitness	Kings Cross	(02) 9356 2555
Beaton Park Leisure Centre	Gwynneville	(02) 4229 6004
BM Sports & Aquatic Ltd	Katoomba	(02) 4782 1748
Body Express	Bondi Beach	(02) 9365 6155
Body Shape Female Fitness Centre	Eastwood	(02) 9907 3642
Bodyheat Health & Fitness Centre	Oatley	(02) 9580 8855
Bodysports	Granville	(02) 9637 8377
Bowral Health Club	Bowral	(02) 4862 5322
Canterbury Aquatic & Fitness Centre	Canterbury	(02) 9789 9303
City Fit Fitness Club	Bathurst	(02) 6331 4344
Club 2000	Castle Hill	(02) 9634 4800
Club Revive	Lithgow	(02) 6353 1272
Come Alive Health & Fitness Centre	Batemans Bay	(02) 4472 5938
Cronulla Fitness Club	Cronulla	(02) 9544 1944
EFM FHF Rydalmere	Rydalmere	0438 642 794
Ettalong Beach Fitness City	Ettalong Beach	(02) 4341 3370
FEKALA Health & Fitness	Bulahdelah	(02) 4997 4454
Fernwood Female Fitness	Parramatta	(02) 9806 0202
	Sydney	(02) 9262 6966

	Haberfield	(02) 9798 8788
	Wollongong	(02) 4226 6162
Fitbodz	Burwood	(02) 9745 2122
Fitness 2000	Erina	(02) 4367 7922
Fitness Edge	West Ryde	(02) 9808 7633
Fitness First	Sydney	(02) 9232 7333
	Bondi Junction	(02) 9389 3999
	Campbelltown	(02) 9620 8838
	Carlingford	(02) 9872 7666
	Dee Why	(02) 9939 3777
	Mosman	(02) 9960 3600
	Randwick	(02) 9326 7800
	St Leonards	(02) 9906 5997
	Sylvania	(02) 9522 4155
	Wollongong	(02) 4229 8884
Fitness Network	Surry Hills	(02) 9211 2799
Fitness Perfection Health	Orange	(02) 6362 6195
& Fitness Club		
Fitness to Perfection	Sydney	(02) 9247 1484
Five Dock Health & Squash	Five Dock	(02) 9713 2344
4 in 1 Fitness	Wyoming	(02) 4328 2244
Gladesville Fitness Centre	Gladesville	(02) 9879 4122
Griffith Indoor Recreation	Griffith	(02) 6962 6666
Harbour Health & Fitness	Coffs Harbour	(02) 6651 1172
Headquarters Fitness Centre	Sydney	(02) 9223 8144
Health Mates Fitness Centre	Revesby	(02) 9792 0726
Health Oasis	Brighton Le Sands	(02) 9567 5130
Healthy Business	North Ryde	(02) 9878 8500
Hiscoes Fitness Centre	Surry Hills	(02) 9699 9222
Howzat Fitness Club	Cooks Hill	(02) 4926 4488
In Shape Health & Fitness Centre	Kensington	(02) 9662 6154
Jackpots Health & Fitness Club	Harbord	(02) 9938 7658
King George V Recreation Centre	Sydney	(02) 9244 3607
Ladies Sanctuary	Gordon	(02) 9418 4988
Lakeside Leisure Centre	Kanahooka	(02) 4261 3693

Lane Cove Fitness	Lane Cove	(02) 9418 9675
Lean & Fit Health Club	Blacktown	(02) 9621 3777
Lean & Fit Health Club	Blacktown	(02) 9830 0677
Leeton Fitness Centre	Leeton	(02) 6953 8133
Leichhardt Park Aquatic Centre	Leichhardt	(02) 9555 8344
Lifestyle Centres in Penrith	Penrith	(02) 4733 3933
Living Well	North Sydney	(02) 9956 5533
	Castle Hill	(02) 9899 4299
Michael Wenden Aquatic & Recreation	Miller	(02) 9607 6598
Millennium Fitness & Lifestyle Centre (*incl. exercise classes for the elderly*)	Waitara	(02) 9987 4277
Mosman Gym	Mosman	(02) 9968 2387
Mounties Fitness Centre	Mt Pritchard	(02) 9610 0300
Newtown Gym	Newtown	(02) 9519 6969
No 1 Martin Place – The Health Club	Sydney City	(02) 9232 1500
NSOP – Lane 9 Gymnasium	South Milsons	(02) 9936 8368
Orange Central Fitness	Orange	(02) 6362 9464
Over Forty Fitness	Mosman	(02) 9960 6660
Prairiewood Leisure Centre	Prairiewood	(02) 9757 2433
ReGenesis	Double Bay	(02) 9363 0376
Ripples Leisure Centre	St Marys	(02) 9833 3000
Roselands Fitness and Squash	Roselands	(02) 9750 4044
Sea Eagles Fitness	Brookvale	(02) 9907 5757
Solar Springs Health & Fitness	Bundanoon	(02) 4883 6027
Sport UNE	Armidale	(02) 6773 2783
Sutherland Leisure Centre	Sutherland	(02) 9545 2400
Sydney International Aquatic Centre	Homebush Bay	(02) 9752 3666
Sydney University Sports Union	University of Sydney	(02) 9351 4960
The Arena Sports Centre	University of Sydney	(02) 9351 8106
The Forum Sports & Aquatic Centre	Callaghan	(02) 4921 7001
The Gym	North Nowra	(02) 4421 0587
The Ladies Sanctuary	Miranda	(02) 9540 4312
The Rock Gym & Spa	Sydney	(02) 9287 4667
Total Planet Fitness	Lambton	(02) 4956 2144

University of NSW	Kensington	(02) 9385 6035
Viking Aquatic & Fitness Centre	Elermore Vale	(02) 4951 3280
Village Fitness Leura	Leura	(02) 4784 2163
Vince & Roz's Fitness World	West Ryde	(02) 9809 2271
Vital Fitness Club	Pennant Hills	(02) 9875 2788
Wests Fitness Centre	New Lambton	(02) 4935 1281
Wests Leagues Health & Fitness	Keiraville	(02) 4271 6890
Willoughby Leisure Centre	Willoughby	(02) 9958 5799

NORTHERN TERRITORY

NAME	SUBURB	PHONE
Carlton Fitness Centre	Darwin City Centre	(08) 8980 0855
Time Out	Darwin City Centre	(08) 8941 8711
Bay Fitness	Cullen Bay	0401 324 389

QUEENSLAND

NAME	SUBURB	PHONE
Alive Gym & Fitness	Strathpine	(07) 3205 3676
Archers Family Fitness Centre	Southport	(07) 5532 5580
Ashgrove Body Designers	Ashgrove	(07) 3366 7706
Australian Crawl Fitness Club	Burpengary	(07) 5431 3507
Beaches Fitness Centre	Smithfield	(07) 4055 6050
Blackwater Fitness Centre	Bluff	(07) 4982 6633
Body Balance Health Club	Mount Isa	(07) 4743 4278
Bodyshop Health & Fitness	Rockhampton	(07) 4928 0333
Bodyworks Health & Fitness (Southside)	Salisbury	(07) 3277 8133
Camp Hill—Carina Welfare Association	Carina	(07) 3398 2107
Central Fitness	Cairns	(07) 4041 2290
City Fitness Centre	Bundaberg	(07) 4152 8566
City Fitness Health Club	Mackay	(07) 4957 8269
Clark's Lifestyle Centre	Tarragindi	(07) 3848 5949
Club Arana	Arana Hills	(07) 3354 2800
Club BJ	Macgregor	(07) 3343 5711

e-Fitness	Bulimba	(07) 3221 7066
Femnasium	Mt Pleasant	(07) 4942 6600
Fit Zone	Runaway Bay	(07) 3852 2755
Fitlink Studio 100	Coorparoo	(07) 3393 0977
Fitness Direct Health Studio	Maroochydore	(07) 5478 1700
Fitness 'n' Motion Health Centre	Morayfield	(07) 5428 2088
Fitness Works	Toowoomba	(07) 4632 7387
Green Apple Gymnasium	Bald Hills	(07) 3261 1249
Healthworks @ Norman Park	Norman Park	(07) 3899 1205
Healthworks Bardon	Bardon	(07) 3366 3511
Healthworks Everton Hills	Everton Hills	(07) 3353 2222
Healthworks Everton Hills	Everton Hills	(07) 3353 3455
Healthworks Hendra	Hendra	(07) 3868 1992
Healthworks on the River	Teneriffe	(07) 3216 1055
Hibiscus Health & Fitness Club	Upper Mt Gravatt	(07) 3403 7564
Highfields Health & Fitness Centre	Toowoomba	(07) 4630 8966
Ipswich Fitness	Ipswich	(07) 3812 1778
Kirwan Fitness	Kirwan	(07) 4773 5244
Living Well Brisbane	Brisbane	(07) 3210 0006
Logan's Hero's	Brown Plains	(07) 3800 7933
Maryborough Fitness, Health and Bodyworks	Maryborough	(07) 4121 6225
Megasports	Browns Plains	(07) 3806 7200
Morningside Fitness	Morningside	(07) 3899 2626
Movements Fitness Centre	Buranda	(07) 3891 6746
Noosa Fitness	Noosa Heads	(07) 5447 3040
Olympus Lifestyle Centre (*formerly Atlantis*)	Alexandra Hills	(07) 3824 0444
QUT Fitness Centre	Brisbane	(07) 3864 1678
QUT Fitness Centre	Brisbane	(07) 3864 1685
Rehabilitation Dynamics	Milton	(07) 3870 5222
Rhonda's Fitness For Ladies	Currajong	(07) 4779 6177
Rothbury Health & Lifestyle Connection	Brisbane	(07) 3220 0130
Sanctuary Cove Recreation Club	Sanctuary Cove	(07) 5577 6083

Shelby's Fun & Fitness Centre	Margate	(07) 3283 8004
Sleeman Health & Fitness Club	Chandler	(07) 3403 9611
Solutions Health & Fitrness Club	North Mackay	(07) 4951 3473
Spirit of Success Health & Fitness Club	Redcliffe	(07) 3883 2800
Sportsmotion	Graceville	(07) 3808 3433
Sportsworld Fitness Centre	Bayview Heights	(07) 4051 2863
Starbodies Healthy Life Centre	Mt Pleasant	(07) 4942 6600
Suncoast Fitness (Kawana)	Kawana	(07) 5493 5933
Suncoast Fitness (Maroochydore)	Maroochydore	(07) 5443 1870
Tropical Bodies Healthy Life Centre	Townsville	(07) 4772 0773
Warwick Indoor Rec. & Aquatic Centre	Warwick	(07) 4661 7955
Workout Indooroopilly	Indooroopilly	(07) 3878 2367
World Fitness Toowoomba	Hendra	(07) 4638 3700
Yaralla Sports Club Inc. Fitness Centre	Gladstone	(07) 4972 2044
YMCA of Brisbane	Roma Street, Brisbane	(07) 3308 0738
YMCA of Bundaberg	Bundaberg	(07) 4152 7178
Other gyms (*with a particular emphasis on older people*) include:		
EFM	Acacia Ridge	0416 246 957
	Albion	0416 246 957
	Bullivants	0411 191 088
Queensland Keep Fit Association	Gympie	(07) 5482 2897
South Bank Fitness Club	South Brisbane	(07) 3844 7111

SOUTH AUSTRALIA

(*Selected list—not necessarily affiliated with Fitness SA*)

NAME	SUBURB	PHONE
Centre for Physical Activity in Aging	Northfield	(08) 8222 1891
EFM	Head Office	0411 744 788
	Burnside	0411 744 800
	Adelaide City	0413 431 403
	FHF Salisbury	0438 250 725
	FHF Underdale	0411 744 788
	Glenelg/Kingswood	0411 743 280
	Santos	0413 706 977

	Stirling	0419 806 430
	Unley	0411 424 304
	Walkerville	0416 153 877
	Womens' and Children's Hospital	0403 049 073
	West Lakes	0411 743 280
	WMC	0416 153 877
Fernwood Female Fitness Centre	Myer Centre Rundle Mall	(08) 8410 0078
	Tranmere	(08) 8332 2966
Fitness on the Park	North Adelaide	(08) 8267 1887
Perfect Fit Health Centres	Burnside	(08) 8364 2933
	Mitcham	(08) 8272 2266
	Glenelg	(08) 8295 8488
	McLaren Vale	(08) 8323 8044
	Modbury	(08) 8396 7333
	Royal Park	(08) 8241 0444
Pro Fitness	Salisbury Plain	(08) 8258 4542
Xclusive Personal Training (caters for older and people with disabilities)	Flinders St, Adelaide	1300 659 900

TASMANIA

NAME	SUBURB	PHONE
All Aerobics	Hobart	(03) 6234 4700
Bayside Fitness	Burnie	(03) 6431 9422
Bethesda Swim Centre	Brighton	(03) 6268 0860
Bodyworks Sports Fitness Centre	Wynyard	(03) 6442 2454
Cazaly Club Fitness	Hobart	(03) 6234 6599
Clarence Police & Citizens Club	Bellerive	(03) 6230 2832
Clarence Swim Centre	Montagu Bay	(03) 6244 2294
Club Salamanca	Battery	(03) 6224 1941
Derwent Valley Swim & Gym Centre	New Norfolk	(03) 6261 4814
Devonport Squash & Recreation Centre	Devonport	(03) 6424 4109
Every Body Fitness	Launceston	(03) 6343 5366
Excel Fitness Studio	Devonport	(03) 6424 5313

Fernwood Female Fitness	Hobart	(03) 6231 1107
	Launceston	(03) 6334 2559
Friends Health & Fitness	North	(03) 6234 2949
Fully Integrated Training	Sandy Bay	(03) 6221 1675
Health & Fitness World	Launceston	(03) 6331 3133
Health & Fitness World	Glenorchy	(03) 6272 4849
Healthglo Fitness Centre	Burnie	(03) 6431 4708
Hobart Police & Citizens Youth Club	Hobart	(03) 6230 2246
Kingborough Sports Centre	Kingston	(03) 6211 8266
Oceana Health & Fitness	Mornington	(03) 6244 6999
Personal Training Fitness Studio	Launceston	(03) 6334 7348
Police Citizens Youth Club	Launceston	(03) 6344 2411
Tattersall's Hobart Aquatic Centre	Hobart	(03) 6222 6999
Templar Squash & Fitness Centre	Devonport	(03) 6427 8540
Theogenes Health & Squash Centre	Launceston	(03) 6331 7399
Ulverstone Recreation Centre	Ulverstone	(03) 6425 6533
Uni of Tas Sports & Recreation Centre	Hobart	(03) 6226 2084
Unitas Consulting Limited	Hobart	(03) 6226 2092
YMCA	Glenorchy	(03) 6272 8077
YMCA Community Centre	Kings Meadows	(03) 6344 3844

VICTORIA

NAME	SUBURB	PHONE
A1 Fitness Club (*South Pacific*)	Moorabbin	(03) 9551 9000
A1 Fitness Club (*South Pacific*)	Richmond	(03) 9427 8994
Action Leisure Centre	Warrnambool	(03) 5562 5050
Adrenalin Health Club	Preston	(03) 9478 1820
API Fitness Centre	Melbourne	(03) 8626 1388
Beach House Fitness Club	Chelsea	(03) 9773 2988
Beach House Womens Fitness	Bentleigh	(03) 9576 5557
Body Image	Hoppers Crossing	(03) 9749 6422
Body World	Balaclava	(03) 9527 7966
	Camberwell	(03) 9882 2201
Bodytrim Health Fitness Centre	Leongatha	(03) 5662 3058
Bodywork Health and Fitness Club	Bulleen	(03) 9850 7000

Boronia Busy Bodies	Boronia	(03) 9762 2222
Brimbank—St Albans Leisure Centre	St Albans	(03) 9367 7899
Brimbank—Sunshine Swim	Sunshine	(03) 9311 5177
& Leisure Centre		
Century Fitness Club	Melbourne	(03) 9329 2100
Church Street Health & Fitness	Brighton	(03) 9593 1066
Colac Squash & Leisure Centre	Colac	(03) 5231 1010
Corporate Health Club—Soffitel	Melbourne	(03) 9654 6144
Corporate Health Club—Grand Mercure	Melbourne	(03) 9621 1577
Cranbourne Fitness & Leisure	Cranbourne	(03) 5996 2055
Dandenong Oasis	Dandenong	(03) 9791 2200
Dandenong Squash and Leisure Centre	Dandenong	(03) 9792 3444
Eastland Fitness Centre	Ringwood	(03) 9870 9355
Equilibrium Health & Fitness	North Melbourne	(03) 9329 4477
	Parkdale	(03) 9587 4464
	Rowville	(03) 9755 7441
Fernwood Female Fitness	Tullamarine	(03) 9330 2712
	Altona North	(03) 9314 2011
	Bendigo	(03) 5441 8008
	Melbourne	(03) 9614 5555
	Hawthorn East	(03) 9804 3600
	Mitcham	(03) 9874 2244
	Narre Warren	(03) 9705 1999
	St Kilda	(03) 9534 8088
	Werribee	(03) 9330 2499
	Greensborough	(03) 9432 5788
Fitness First	Highett	(03) 9532 2898
	Richmond	(03) 9425 9888
Five Star Fitness	Thomastown	(03) 9465 2002
Focus Health & Fitness	Tullamarine	(03) 9338 6418
Freeway Sports Centre	Doveton	(03) 9791 5777
Genesis Health Club	Doncaster	(03) 9848 6111
	Toorak	(03) 9568 1112
	Ringwood	(03) 9870 1666
Greenhouse Fitness Club	Mulgrave	(03) 9547 0722

Horsham City Gym	Horsham	(03) 5382 0423
Hunts Dingley Fitness Club	Dingley	(03) 9551 3022
Hunts Fitness Centre	Fitzroy	(03) 9419 3636
Hyatt—City Club Health & Fitness	Melbourne	(03) 9653 4894
Hyatt—Park Club Health & Day Spa	Melbourne	(03) 9224 1222
Input Fitness	Frankston	(03) 9789 3566
King Club	Cheltenham	(03) 9584 7233
Ladyworks	Hawthorn East	(03) 9882 0006
Lakes Health & Fitness	Taylors Lakes	(03) 9390 9099
Leisure City Health Club	Epping	(03) 9401 2247
Lifestyle Fitness Centre	Brighton	(03) 9592 8022
	Melbourne	(03) 9670 9291
	Forest Hill	(03) 9894 1929
	Frankston	(03) 9781 5533
	Mornington	(03) 5975 6000
	Newport	(03) 9399 1100
	Richmond	(03) 9428 6666
	Bendigo	(03) 5442 1599
	Wheelers Hill	(03) 9561 6933
	Wodonga	(02) 6024 7088
Melbourne City Baths	Melbourne	(03) 9663 5888
Melbourne Fitness Club	Melbourne	(03) 9629 4299
Mt Eliza Squash and Fitness	Mount Eliza	(03) 9787 4442
Ocean View Health Club	Ocean Grove	(03) 5255 2572
Personal Best Fitness Centre	Bayswater	(03) 9720 5556
Premier Health Club	Newtown	(03) 5221 1126
Pulse Wellness Club	Essendon	(03) 9337 3100
Queens Park Health Club	Melbourne	(03) 9804 5855
RANS—Morwell Leisure Centre	Morwell	(03) 5133 9900
RANS—Sanctuary, Staff Gym, Crown Casino	Southbank	(03) 9292 7759
RANS—Windy Hill Fitness Centre	Essendon	(03) 9375 1555
Re-Creation Health Club—Armadale	Armadale	(03) 9509 7622
Reservoir Leisure Centre	Reservoir	(03) 9462 1677
Studio Female Fitness	Sunbury	(03) 9740 7633

The Fitness Hub	Syndal	(03) 9802 1433
The Ridge Health Club	Eltham	(03) 9431 1223
	Melton	(03) 9743 4477
Trackside Sports & Fitness	Hampton	(03) 9597 0579
Virginia Park Health Club	East Bentleigh	(03) 9570 2738
Westgate Health Club	Altona North	(03) 9369 6622
Winning Edge Health Club	Chadstone	(03) 9569 0200
	Balwyn	(03) 9817 4496
Yarra Leisure Services	Clifton Hill	(03) 9205 5522
Zaks Health Club	Prahran	(03) 9525 2944

WESTERN AUSTRALIA

NAME	SUBURB	PHONE
Active 8 Paragon Health and Fitness Club	Perth CBD	(08) 9322 1588
Arena Joondalup	Joondalup	(08) 9300 7171
Bay of Isles	Esperance	(08) 9072 0222
Bayswater Waves	Bayswater	(08) 9276 6538
BC The Body Club	Claremont	(08) 9385 5452
Beatty Park L/C	North Perth	(08) 9273 6080
Belmont Oasis	Belmont	(08) 9277 1022
CBD Health Spa	Perth CBD	(08) 9221 9900
Central TAFE	Northbridge	(08) 9427 5390
City of Gosnells Leisure World	Gosnells	(08) 9493 4399
Complete Fitness	Malaga	(08) 9249 4544
Curtin Recreation Services	Bentley	(08) 9427 2483
Energy Gym	Morley	(08) 9371 8088
Evolution	Victoria Park	(08) 9470 2177
Fitness Express	Morley	(08) 9276 8166
Fremantle Leisure Centre	Fremantle	(08) 9432 9533
Gymcare	Bassendean	(08) 9379 1888
Katanning Leisure	Katanning	(08) 9821 4399
Loftus Recreation Centre	Leederville	(08) 9227 6526
Lords Sports Club	Subiaco	(08) 9381 4777
Melville Recreation Centre	Melville	(08) 9330 9933

Murray District Recreation Centre	Pinjarra	(08) 9531 2000
Park Recreation Centre	Victoria Park	(08) 9362 6066
Renaissance Fitness Centre	Midland	(08) 9274 6144
Selby Health	Osborne Park	(08) 9446 7372
Westin Fitness	Balga	(08) 9342 0111

Workout sheet

DAY	EXERCISE	WEIGHTS	REPS	SETS 1 2 3 4 5 6	NOTES

Bibliography

Aaberg, E., *Resistance Training Instruction: Advanced Principles and Techniques for Fitness Professionals*, Human Kinetics, Champaign, Ill.

Allen, P.R., Denham, R.A. & Swan, A.J., 'Late degenerative changes after meniscectomy', *J Bone Joint Surg*, 1984, 66B, pp. 666–77.

American College of Sports Medicine, *Guidelines for Exercise Testing and Prescription* (6th edn), American College of Sports Medicine, Lippincott Williams & Wilkins, Philadelphia 2000,.

Baur, L.A. 'Obesity: Definitely a growing concern', *Med J Aust*, 2001, 174, pp. 553–4.

Bigos, S.J. & Battie, M.C., 'Industrial low back pain', in S.W. Wiesel, J.N. Weinstein, I.I. Herkowitz et al. (eds), *The Lumbar Spine* (2nd ed), 1996, W.B. Saunders Co, Phildelphia, 1996pp, 1065–105.

Borushek, A. *Pocket Calorie Counter*, Family Health Publications, Perth, 1988,.

Brown, A. McCartney, N. & Sole, D. 'Positive adaptations to weight-lifting training in older adults', *Am J Clin Nutr*, 60, 1994, pp. 167–75.

Campbell, W.W., Crim, M.C., Young, V.R. et al. 'Increased energy requirements and changes in body composition with resistance training in older adults', *Am J Clin Nutr*, 60, 1994, pp. 167–75.

Chard, M.D., Cawston, T.E., Riley, G.P. et al. 'Rotator cuff degeneration and lateral epicondylitis: a comparative histological study', *Ann Rheum Dis*, 53, 1994, pp. 30–4.

Chodzko-Zajko, W.J. 'Physiology of aging and exercise', in R.T. Cotton (ed.), *Exercise for Older Adults*, San Diego, American Council on Exercise, 1998, pp. 2–23.

Clark, J. 'Older adult exercise techniques', in R.T. Cotton (ed), *Exercise for Older Adults*, San Diego, American Council on Exercise, 1998, pp. 130–81.

Cleland, L.G. & James, M.J., 'Fish oil and RA: anti-inflammatory and collateral health benefits', *J Rheumatol*, 27, 2000, pp. 2305–7.

Cleland, L.G. & James, M.J. 'Omega 3 and a health diet', *Arthritis Today*, Spring, 2000, pp. 18–21.

Commachio, A., personal communication.

Commonwealth Department of Health and Aged Care (DHAC), National Physical Activity Guidelines for Australians, Canberra, 1999.

Cooper, C., McAlindon, T., Snow, S. et al. 'Mechanical and constitutional risk factors for symptomatic knee OA: differences between mecia tibiofemoral and patellofemoral disease', *J Rheumatol*, 21, 1994, pp. 307–13.

Cotton R.T. (ed.) *Exercise for Older Adults* (1st edn), San Diego, ACE, 1998.

Cotton, R.T. 'Testing and evaluation', in American Council on Exercise, *Personal Trainer Manual* (2nd edn), San Diego, ACE, 1996.

Cottreau, C.M., Ness, R.B. & Kriska, A.M. 'Physical activity and reduced risk of ovarian cancer', *Obstetrics and Gynaecology*, 96, 2000, pp. 609–14.

Davis, S.R., Burger, H.G., Bass, S.L. et al. 'Identifying and promoting the specific nutrition and physical activity needs of women aged 40 and over', *Med J Aust*, 173, pp. (Suppl), 2000, pp. S89–S112.

Després, J.P., Pouliot, M.C., Moorjami, S. et al. 'Loss of abdominal fat and metabolic response to exercise training in obese women', *Am J Physiol*, 261, 1991, pp. E159–E167.

Durrington, P.N. Bhatnager, D., Mackness, M.I. et al. 'An omega-3 polyunsaturated fatty acid concentrate administered for one year decreased triglycerides in simvastatin treated patients with coronary heart disease and persisting hypertriglyceridaemia', *J Heart*, 85, 2001, pp. 544–8.

Eckel, R.H. & Krauss, R.M., American Heart Association call to action: obesity as a major risk factor for coronary heart disease', AHA Nutrition Committee, *Circulation*, 97, 1998, pp. 2099–100.

Eckersley, R.M. 'Losing the battle of the bulge: causes and consequences of increasing obesity', *Med J Aust*, 174, 2001, pp. 590–2.

Engels, H.J., Smith, C.R. & Wirth, J.C., 'Metabolic and haemodynamic responses to walking with shoulder-worn exercise weights: a brief report', *Clin J Sports Med*, 5, 1995, pp. 171–4.

Erdman, J.W. Jr, 'Soy protein and cardiovascular disease: a statement for health care professionals from the Nutrition Committee of the AHA', *Circulation*, 102, 2000, pp. 2555–9.

Evans, W.J. 'Reversing sarcopenia: how weight training can build strength and vitality', *Geriatrics*, 51, 1996, pp. 51–8.

Feldmann, S. 'Exercise for the person with rheumatoid arthritis', in R.W. Chang (ed.), *Rehabilitation in Persons with Rheumatoid Arthritis*, Gaithersburg, Md, Aspen, 1996.

Fiatarone, M.A., Marks, E.C. Ryan, N.D. et al. 'High-intensity strength training in nonagenarians', *JAMA*, 263, 1990, pp. 3029–34.

Fiatarone, M.A. & Evans, W.J. 'The etiology and reversibility of muscle dysfunction in the elderly', *J Gerontol*, 48, 1993, pp. 77–83.

Fiatarone, M.A., Ding, W, Manfredi, T. J. et al. 'Insulin-like growth factor I in skeletal muscle after weight-lifting exercise in frail elders', *Am J Physiol*, 277, 1999, pp. 135–43.

Fletcher, G.F, Blair, S.N., Blumenthal, J. et al. 'Statement on exercise: benefits and recommendations for physical activity programs for all Americans: a statement for health professionals by the Committee on Exercise and Cardiac Rehabilitation of the Council on Clinical Cardiology', in American Health Association, *Circulation*, 86, 1992, pp. 340–44.

Fogelholm, M. 2000 Pre-Olympic Congress, International Congress on Sports Medicine, Sports Medicine and Physical Medicine, Brisbane, 7–12 September 2000.

Hadler, N.M. 'Osteoarthritis as a public health problem', *Clin Rheum Dis*, 11, 1985, pp. 175–85.

Hakkinen, A. & Sokka, T. et al. 'A randomised two-year study of the effects of dynamic strength training on muscle strength, disease activity, functional capacity and bone mineral density in early rheumatoid arthritis', *Arthritis Rheum*, 44, 2001, pp. 515–22.

Hamilton-Craig, I. *Cholesterol Control*, William Heinemann, 1987.

Heikkinen, E., Suominen, H., Era, P. et al. 'Variations in aging parameters, their sources, and possibilities of predicting physiological age', in A.K. Balin (ed.), *Practical Handbook of Human Biologic Age Determination*, CRC Press, New York, 1994, pp. 71–92.

Hult, L. 'Cervical, dorsal and lumbar spine syndromes: a field investigation of a non-selected material of 1200 workers in different occupations with special reference to disc degeneration and so-called muscular rheumatism', *Acta Orthop Scand*, Supp 17, 1954, pp. 1–102.

Humphries, B., Newton, R.U., Bronks, R. et al. 'Effective exercise intensity on bone density, strength and calcium turnover in older women', *Med Sci Sports Exercise*, 32, 2000, pp. 1043–50.

Iso, H., Rexrode, K.M, Stampfer, M.J. et al. 'Intake of fish and omega-3 fatty acids and risk of stroke in women', *JAMA*, 285, 2001, pp. 304–12.

James, M.J. & Cleland, L.G. 'Fats and oils: the facts', http://wwwl.goldencanola.com.au

Kane, R., Oslander, J. and Abrass, I., *Essentials of Clinical Geriatrics* (2nd edn), McGraw-Hill, Information Services Co, New York, 1989.

Katan, M.B., 'Effect of low-fat diets on plasma high-density lipoprotein concentrations', *Am J Clin Nutr*, 67, Suppl S73–S76, 1998.

Krauss, R.M., Winston, M., Fletcher, R.N. et al. 'Obesity: impact of cardiovascular disease', *Circulation*, 98, 1998, pp. 1472–6.

Laukkanenen, J.A., Lakka, T.A. et al. 'Cardiovascular fitness as a predictor of mortality in men', *Arch Intern Med*, 26, 161(6), 2001, pp. 825–31.

Lawrence, J.S., 'Disc degeneration: its frequency and relationship to symptoms', *Ann Rheum Dis*, 28, 1969, pp. 121–37.

Lawrence, J.S., Bremner, J.M. & Beir, F. 'Osteoarthritis: prevalence in the population and relationship between symptoms and x-ray changes', *Ann Rheum Dis*, 25, 1966, pp. 1–23.

Lee, I.M, Sesso, H.D. & Paffenburger, R.S. Jr, 'Physical activity and coronary artery disease risk in men: does the duration of exercise episodes predict risk?', *Circulation*, 102, 2000, pp. 981–6.

Lequesne, M.G., Dang, N. & Lane, N.E., 'Sport practice in osteoarthritis of the limbs', *Osteoarthritis Cartilage*, 5, 1997, pp. 75–86.

McAlindon, T.E., Cooper, C., Kirwan, F.R. et al. 'Determinants in disability in osteoarthritis of the knee', *Ann Rheum Dis*, 52, 1993, pp. 258–62.

Magora, A. 'Investigation of the relation between low-back pain and occupation, v. psychological aspects', *Scand J Rehab Med*, 5, 1973, pp. 191–6.

Martinsen, E.W., Medhus, A. & Sandvik, L., 'Effects of aerobic exercise on depression: a controlled study', *BMJ*, 291, 1985, p. 109.

Martinson, B.C., O'Connor, P.J. & Pronk, N.P., 'Physical inactivity and short-term all-cause mortality in adults with chronic disease', *Arch Intern Med*, 14, 161(9), 2001, pp. 1173–80.

Morgan, A.L., Ellison, J.D., Chandler, M.P. et al. 'The supplemental benefits of strength training for aerobically active postmenopausal women', *J Aging and Phys Act*, 3, 1995, pp. 332–9.

Morgan, T., personal communication.

Morris, M.C., Sacks, F. & Rosner, B., 'Does fish oil lower blood pressure? A meta-analysis of controlled trials', *Circulation*, 88, 1993, pp. 523–33.

Moul, J.L., Goldman, B. & Warren, B., 'Physical activity and cognitive performance in the older population', *J Aging Phys Act*, 2, 1995, pp. 135–144.
National Physical Activity Guidelines for Australians, Commonwealth Department of Health and Aged Care (DHAC), Canberra, 1999.

Nelson, M.E. & Wernick, S. *Strong Women Stay Slim*, Lothian, Melbourne, 1998.

Noakes, M., personal communication.

Noakes, M., Clifton, P. & McMurchie, T. 'The role of diet in cardiovascular health: a review of the evidence', *Aust J Nutr Diet*, 56 (3 Suppl), 1999, pp. S3–S22.

Petersson, C.J., 'Degeneration of the acromioclavicular joint', *Acta Orthop Scand*, 54, 1983, pp. 434–8.

Phillips, B. & D'Orso, M. *Body for Life*, HarperCollins, New York, 1999.

Pollock, M.L., Gaesser, G.A., Butcher, J.D. et al. 'The recommended quantity and quality of exercise for developing and maintaining cardiorespiratory and muscular fitness, and flexibility in healthy adults', *Med Sci Sports Exerc*, 30, 1998, pp. 975–91.

Pollock, M.L., Graves, J.E., Stewart, D.L. et al. 'Exercise training and prescription for the elderly', *Southern Medical Journal*, 87, 1994, pp. S88–S95.

Pollock, M.L., Leggett, S.H., Graves, J.E. et al. 'Effect of resistance training on lumbar extension strength', *Am J Sports Med*, 17, 1989, pp. 624–9.

Powell, K.E. et al. 'Physical activity and the incedence of coronary heart disease', *Annual Review Public Health*, 8, 1987, pp. 253–87.

Rimmer, J.H. 'Common health challenges faced by older adults', in R.T. Cotton (ed.), *Exercise for Older Adults* (1st edn), American Council on Exercise, San Diego, CA, 1998.

Ross, R., Dagnone, D., Jones, P.J. et al. 'Reduction in obesity and related co-morbid conditions after diet-induced or exercise-induced weight loss: a randomised controlled trial', *Ann Intern Med*, 133, 2000, pp. 92–103.

Salmeron, J., Hu, F.B. et al. 'Dietary fat intake and risk of type 2 diabetes in women', *Am J Clin Nutr*, 73(6), June 2001, pp. 1019–26.

Schneiter, P., Di Vetta, V. Jequier, E. et al. 'The effect of physical exercise on glycogen turnover and net substrate utilisation according to the nutritional state', *Am J Physiol*, 269, 1995, pp. 1031–6.

Siscovick, D.S., Weiss, N.S., Fletcher, R.H. et al. 'The incidence of primary cardia arrest during vigorous exercise', *N Engl J Med*, 311, 1984, pp. 874–7.

Spirduso, W. & Macrae, P.G. 'Motor performance and aging', in J. Birren, J. Lubbon, R. Cichowlas & D. Deutchman (eds), *Handbook of the Psychology of Aging* (3rd edn), Academic Press, San Diego, 1990.

Spirduso, W.W., *Physical Dimensions of Aging*, Human Kinetics Pub., Champaign, Ill, 1995.

Stanton, R. 'Exercise judgement', *Australian Doctor*, 6 October 2000, pp. 55–6.

Stanton, R. Exercise Judgement: a report on the 2000 Pre-Olympic Congress, International Congress on Sports Science, Sports Medicine and Physical Medicine, Brisbane, 7–12 September 2000, *Australian Doctor*, 6 October 2000, pp. 55–6.

Terry, P., Lichtenstein, P. et al. 'Fatty fish consumption and risk of prostate cancer', *Lancet*, 357 (9270), 2 June 2000, pp. 1764–66.

Terry, P., Giovannucci, E. et al. 'Fruit, vegetables, dietary fiber, and risk of colorectal cancer', *J Natl Cancer Inst*, 4, 93(7), 2001, pp. 525–33.

Thompson, S. & Hoekengas, J. 'Understanding and motivating older adults', in R.T. Cotton, *Exercise for Older Adults* (1st edn), American Council on Exercise, San Diego, CA, 1998.

Topping, D.L. & Bird, A.R., 'Foods, nutrients and digestive health', Aust J Nutr Diet, 56 (3 Suppl), 1999, pp. S22–S34.

US Department of Health and Human Services, *Physical Activity and Health: A Report of the Surgeon General*, US Department of Health and Human Services, Centers for Disease Control and Prevention, National Centre for Chronic Disease Prevention and Health Promotion and the Presidentís Council on Physical Fitness and Sports, Atlanta, GA, 1996.

Volker, D., Fitzgerald, P., Major, G. et al. 'Efficacy of fish oil concentrate in the treatment of rheumatoid arthritis', *J Rheumatol*, 27, 2000, pp. 2343–6.

Westcott, W.L. & Baechle, T.R., *Strength Training Past 50*, Human Kinetics, Champaign, Ill, 1998.

Worrell, T.W., Smith, T.W. & Winegardner, J. 'Effect of hamstring stretching on hamstring muscle performance', *J Orth & Sports Phys Ther*, 20, 1994, pp. 154–9.

Index